EVERYWOMAN

EVERYWOMAN

and Her Body

Derek Llewellyn-Jones, M.D.

TAPLINGER PUBLISHING COMPANY
New York

First published in the United States in 1971 by
TAPLINGER PUBLISHING CO., INC.
New York, New York

International Standard Book Number 0-8008-2535-7

Library of Congress Catalog Card Number 72-153672

Printed in Great Britain

CONTENTS

ILLUSTRATIONS

PREFACE

Modern woman is considerably interested in herself. She is anxious to know about the changes which occur in her body each month. She wants to know about contraceptive techniques. She is involved increasingly in her own care during pregnancy, and seems increasingly to desire to know what happens during pregnancy and childbirth. She is even more concerned with her sexual role in marriage.

It is a most healthy development, and to meet this demand for information, a constant stream of articles appear in women's magazines. These articles are supplemented by a large number of books.

Two main approaches are used by the authors of these articles and books. In the first the author adopts the physiological-medical attitude, and explains his points precisely in clinical language; for example, '. . . at this point the penis is introduced into the hyperaemic vagina, clitoral stimulation being enhanced by counter-pressure and concomitant friction'. In the second approach purple prose and mystical passion pervade the pages, for example '. . . at moments like this an intense feeling of deep longing enwraps the girl. The stars stop in their courses, the moon hangs silvered in the branches, music falls from the air, and a wondrous tenderness pervades this delicate moment of sweet passion, when a woman soars in an ecstasy all her own'.

Both of these approaches have their adherents and their devotees, to judge from the sales of the books! But both miss, to some extent, the point that modern woman is intelligent, interested in her femininity, and adult in her attitudes.

It is with this belief that *Everywoman* has been written. I hope that I have avoided the whirlpool of brusque clinical detail and the rosy romantic rocks of purple prose. I have made an effort to put myself in the position of an intelligent modern woman aged from 17 to 67 who wants to know more about herself, and who would like to have available a book to which she could refer at times in her life which are particularly related to her femininity.

When the book was written, I asked a group of women for their comments and criticisms. Their help has been much appreciated and their names should be recorded, with my sincere thanks: May Kirkby, Nola Clarke, Jennifer Pockley, Hilary Linstead and Dorothy Maher. Even more are my thanks due to my Secretary, Nicola Stemp, who not only typed and retyped the manuscript, but joined the readers and commented most helpfully on the text.

Fig. 7/1, The growth of the world's population, has been redrawn from *Population Bulletin*, **18**, 1, 1962 with their kind permission. I should also like to thank the Ortho Pharmaceutical Corporation, Raritan, N.J. for their permission to reproduce the illustrations of the vaginal diaphragm, Fig. 7/5A, B, C and E. Figs. 9/2 to 9/11 have been redrawn from a series published in *Pregnancy in Anatomical Transparencies* by the Carnation Co. and I am grateful to them for their permission.

Finally, I would dedicate this book to two women – to my wife, Elisabeth, and to our daughter, Deborah. It seems appropriate that a book about women should be dedicated to two women whom I have known and loved for longer, and more closely, than any others.

DEREK LLEWELLYN-JONES
Sydney, 1971

CHAPTER 1

A woman is different

Even in these days of unisex fashions, the distinction between a man and a woman is relatively easy! Not only does a woman's psychological make-up differ from that of a man–although exactly how much of this is due to the prevailing cultural attitudes is not clear–but quite obviously she is anatomically different. Amongst Western communities, the breast has a unique sexual symbolism, and even if fashion diminishes its rotundity, the hemispherical mammary glands are a potent attraction for the male eye. In more primitive communities, where breasts are habitually exposed, they have no sexual connotation, being considered for what they are–a source of nourishment for the infant.

The more specific anatomical differences are of the genital organs. The proud male external genitals–the penis and the testicles–are absent in woman, a fact which suggested to Freud that many of woman's sexual problems related to an envy for the absent penis and a complex that the testicles had been castrated. Woman was therefore a mutilated male, and inferior to man. Freud was in fact more than unfair to women, and considerably confused about women, possibly because of his own upbringing in a traditional Jewish middle-class family. He held that woman had a smaller intellectual capacity, a far greater vanity, a constitutional passivity, a weaker sexuality, and a greater disposition to neurosis. At the same time, he considered her enigmatic, her femininity a complicated process, her psychology involved. Studies over the past half-century have shown that Freud's view of woman as an inferior, mutilated male is incorrect, and his assessment of her inferiority and her instability is more an indictment of the cultural environment in which she is brought up, than of her inherited make-up. In other words, a woman behaves in a certain way because she is brought up to believe that society expects her to behave in that way. This does not imply that she is weaker or inferior to a man, even if both are brought up by society to believe this. Indeed, longevity studies show that the female is stronger than the male, less likely to be aborted when in her mother's womb, more likely to be born alive, less likely to succumb to infection in the first years of life, and more likely to live beyond the age of 65.

Given the opportunity, a woman can succeed in most activities as well as a man, but in one activity she is unique. The human female is a mammal. She carries her infant in the womb until it is sufficiently well developed to survive, or at least to suck, she suckles it and cares for it. This process of internal development of the infant is only possible because the womb–or uterus–is in a protected position, enclosed by the strong bones of the female pelvis.

Although the uterus is central to the anatomical difference between male and female, the most obvious differences are those of the external genitalia, which will be described first. After that, the internal genital organs, the vagina, the uterus, the oviducts and the ovaries will be described, for unless a woman has some idea of her anatomy much of what follows in this book will be less easily understood.

THE EXTERNAL GENITALIA IN THE FEMALE

The anatomical name for the area of the external genitalia in the female is the *vulva*. It is made up of several structures which surround the entrance to the vagina, and each of which has its own separate function (Fig. **1/1**). The *labia majora* (or the large lips of the vagina) are two large folds of skin which contain sweat glands and hair follicles embedded in fat. The size of the labia majora varies considerably. In infancy and in old age they are small, and the fat is not present; in the reproductive years, between puberty and the menopause, they are well filled with fatty tissue. In front (looked at from between the legs), they join together in the pad of fat which surmounts the pelvic bone, and which was called the *'mount of Venus' (mons veneris)* by the ancient anatomists, when they noted that it was most developed in the reproductive years. Both of the labia, and more particularly the mons veneris, are covered with hair, the quantity of which varies from woman to woman. The pubic hair on the abdominal side of the mons veneris terminates in a straight line, whilst in the male the hair stretches upwards in an inverted 'V' to reach

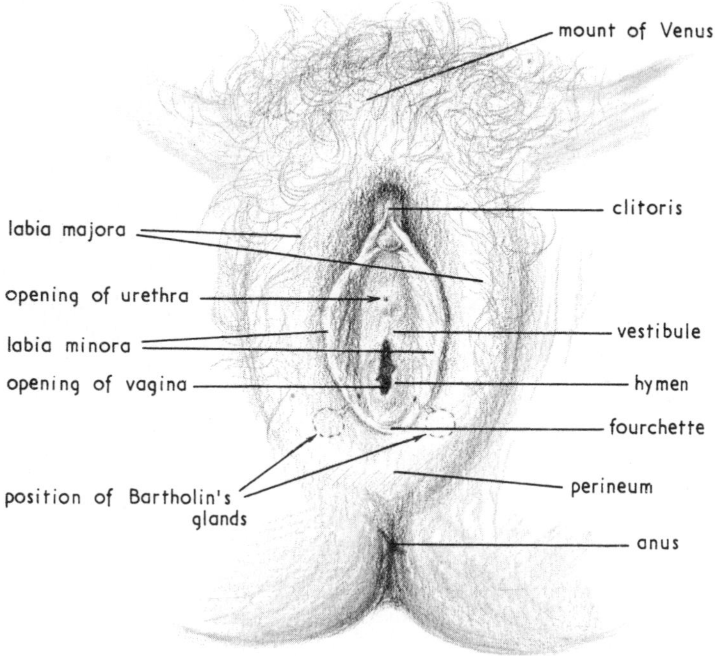

FIG. 1/1. The external genitals in a virgin

the umbilicus (Fig. **1/2**). The inner surfaces of the labia majora are free from hair, and are separated by a small groove from the thin labia minora, which guard the entrance to the vagina.

The *labia minora* (the small lips) are delicate folds of skin which contain little fatty tissue. They vary in size, and it was once believed that large labia minora were due to masturbation, which at that time was considered evil. It is now known that this is nonsense. In front, the labia minora split into two folds, one of which passes over and the other under the *clitoris,* and at the back they join to form the *fourchette,* which is always torn during childbirth. In the reproductive years, the labia minora are hidden by the enlarged labia majora, but in childhood and old age the labia minora appear more prominent because the labia majora are relatively small.

The *clitoris* is the exact female equivalent of the male penis. The fold of the labia minora which passes over it is equivalent to the

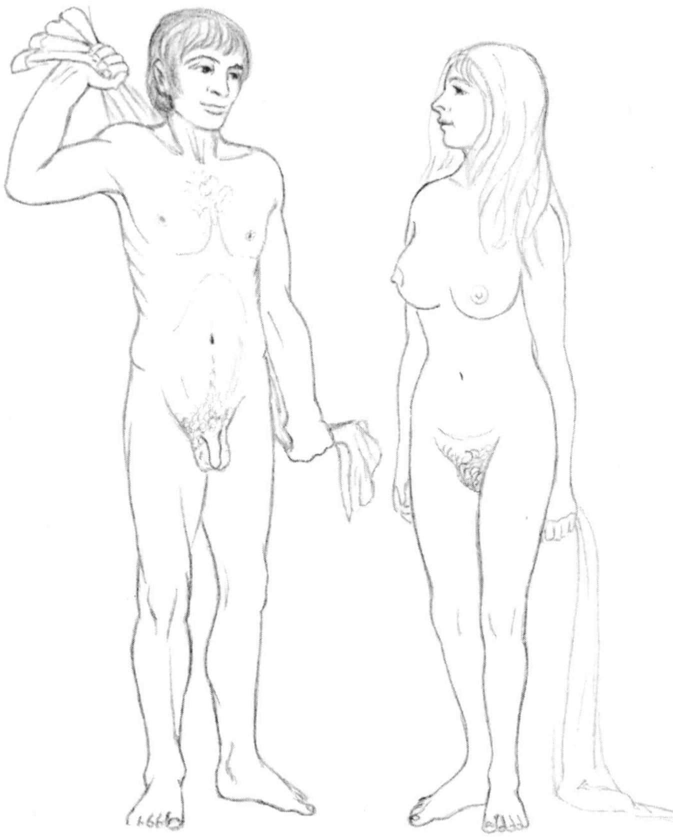

FIG. 1/2. The male and female from the front

male foreskin (prepuce). It covers and protects the clitoris. The fold which passes under it is equivalent to the small band of tissue which joins the pink glans of the penis to the skin which covers it. It is called the *frenulum*. The clitoris is made up of erectile tissue, which fills with blood during sexual excitement. It is extremely sensitive to the touch, and movement of the penis against the clitoris in sexual intercourse, or by gentle stroking with the finger, can lead to orgasm.

The clitoris varies considerably in size, but is usually that of a green pea; as sexual excitement mounts, the clitoris increases in size. Once again this varies considerably between individuals.

The cleft below the clitoris and between the labia minora is called the *vestibule* (or entrance). Just below the clitoris is the external opening of that part of the urinary tract (the *urethra*) which connects the bladder to the outside world. In old women the urethral orifice may stretch, and the lining of the lower part of the urethra may be exposed.

Below the external urethral orifice is the hymen, which surrounds the vaginal orifice. The hymen is a thin incomplete fold of membrane, which has one or more apertures in it. It varies considerably in shape and in elasticity, but is generally stretched or torn during the first attempt at sexual intercourse. The tearing is usually followed by a minute amount of bleeding. In many cultures the rupture of the hymen (also called the maidenhead), and the consequent bleed, was considered a sign that the girl was a virgin at the time of marriage, and the bed was inspected on the morning after the first night of the honeymoon for evidence of blood. Although an 'intact' hymen is considered a sign of virginity, it is not a reliable sign, as in some cases coitus fails to cause a tear, and in others the hymen may have been torn previously by exploring fingers, either of the girl herself or of a consort. The stretching and tearing of the hymen at a first copulation may be painful, particularly if the partners are apprehensive or ignorant of sexual matters. If the couple are well adjusted, the discomfort is minimal. Childbirth causes a much greater tearing of the hymen, and after delivery only a few tags remain. They are called *carunculae myrtiformes* (Fig. **1/3**). Just outside the hymen, still within the vestibule but deep beneath the skin, are two collections of erectile tissue which fill with blood during sexual arousal. Deep in the backward part of the vestibule are two pea-sized glands which also secrete fluid during sexual arousal and moisten the entrance to the vagina, so that the penis may more readily enter it without discomfort. These glands occasionally become infected. They are known as *Bartholin's glands*.

The area of the vulva between the posterior fourchette and the anus, and the muscles which lie under the skin, form a pyramid-shaped wedge of tissue separating the vagina and the rectum. It is called the *perineum*, and is of considerable importance in childbirth.

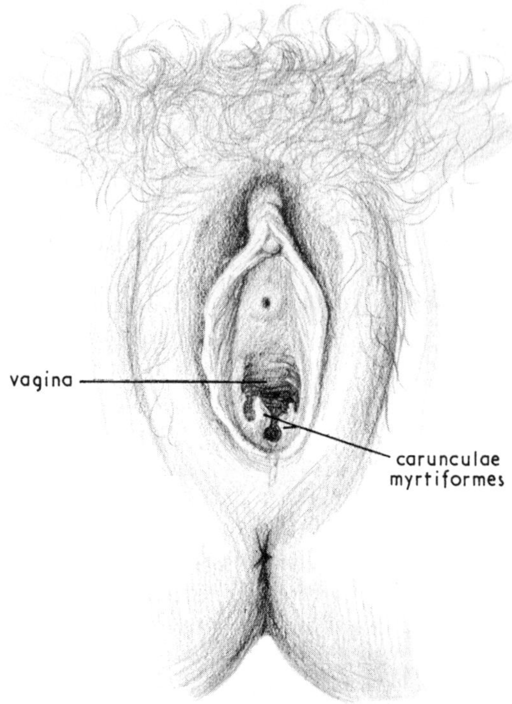

FIG. 1/3. The external genitals in a woman who has had a child

THE INTERNAL GENITAL ORGANS

The *vagina* is a muscular tube which stretches upwards and backwards from the vestibule to reach the uterus. As well as being muscular, it contains a well-developed network of veins which become distended in sexual arousal. Normally the walls of the vagina lie close together, the vagina being a potential cavity which is distended by intravaginal tampons used during menstruation, by the penis at copulation, and during childbirth, when it can stretch very considerably to permit the baby to be born. The vagina is about 9 cm. ($3\frac{3}{4}$ in.) long, and at the upper end the *cervix* (or neck) of the uterus projects into it (Fig. **1/4**). The vagina lies between the bladder

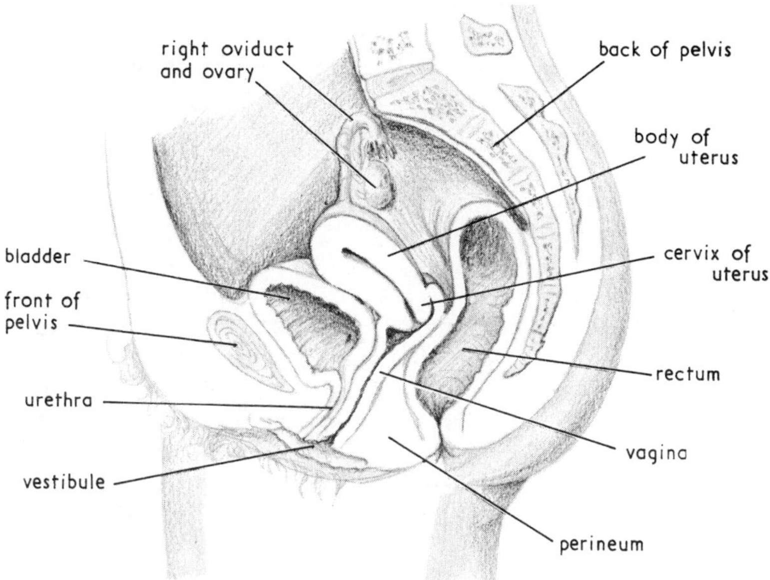

FIG. 1/4. The internal genital organs of the female

in front and the rectum (or back-passage) behind. At the sides it is surrounded and protected by the strong muscles of the floor of the pelvis. Unless the vagina has been damaged, injured or tightened at operation, or has not developed due to an absence of sex hormones, its size is quite adequate for sexual intercourse. The woman who menstruates has a normal-sized vagina, and 'difficulty' at intercourse is not due to her being 'small made'. This is a myth. The cause lies not in the vagina, but in a mental fear of sexual intercourse which leads the woman to tighten the muscles which support the vagina to such an extent that coitus is painful.

The vagina is a remarkable organ. Not only is it capable of great distension, but it keeps itself clean. The cells which form its walls are 30 cells deep, lying on each other like the bricks of a house wall. In the reproductive years, the top layer of cells is constantly being shed into the vagina, where the cells are acted upon by a small bacillus which normally lives there, to produce lactic acid. The lactic acid then kills any contaminating germs which may happen to get into the vagina. Because of this, 'cleansing' vaginal douches, so popular at one time in the U.S.A., are unnecessary. In childhood, the wall of the vagina is thin, and the production of lactic acid does not take place. However this is of little importance, because the vagina is not usually contaminated at this age. In old age, the lining becomes thin once again, and few cells are shed. Because of this, little or no lactic acid is formed, and contaminating germs may grow. This sometimes results in inflammation of the vagina.

The *uterus* is an even more remarkable organ than the vagina. Before pregnancy it is pear-shaped, averages 9 cm. ($3\frac{3}{4}$ in.) in length, 6 cm. ($2\frac{1}{2}$ in.) in width at its widest point, and weighs 60 g. (2 oz.). In pregnancy, it enlarges to weigh 1,000 g. ($2\frac{1}{4}$ lb.), and is able to contain a baby measuring 40 cm. (17 in.) in length. It is able to undergo these changes because of the complex structure of its muscle and its exceptional response to the female sex hormones. The uterus is a hollow, muscular organ, which is located in the middle of the bony pelvis, lying between the bladder in front and the bowel behind (Fig. **1/4**). It is pear-shaped, and its muscular front and back walls bulge into the cavity which is normally narrow and slit-like, until pregnancy occurs. Viewed from in front, the cavity is triangular, and is lined with a special tissue made up of glands in a network of cells. This tissue is called the endometrium, and it undergoes changes during each menstrual cycle. For descriptive purposes, the uterus is divided into an upper part, or *body*, and a lower portion, or *cervix uteri*. The word cervix means neck, so that the 'cervix uteri' means the neck of the womb. The cavity is narrow in the cervix, where it is called the cervical canal; widest in the body of the uterus; and then narrows again towards the cornu (or horn), where the cavity is continuous with the hollow of the Fallopian tube (Fig. **1/5**). The cervix projects into the upper part of the vagina, and is a particular place where cancer sometimes develops. As it is readily accessible for examination, early changes in the cells indicating that cancer may be about to occur can be sought by special methods. This is discussed in more detail in Chapter 20. The lower part of the uterus and the upper part of the cervix are supported by a sling of special tissues, which stretch to the muscles of the pelvic wall in a fan-like manner. These supports may be stretched in childbirth, leading to a

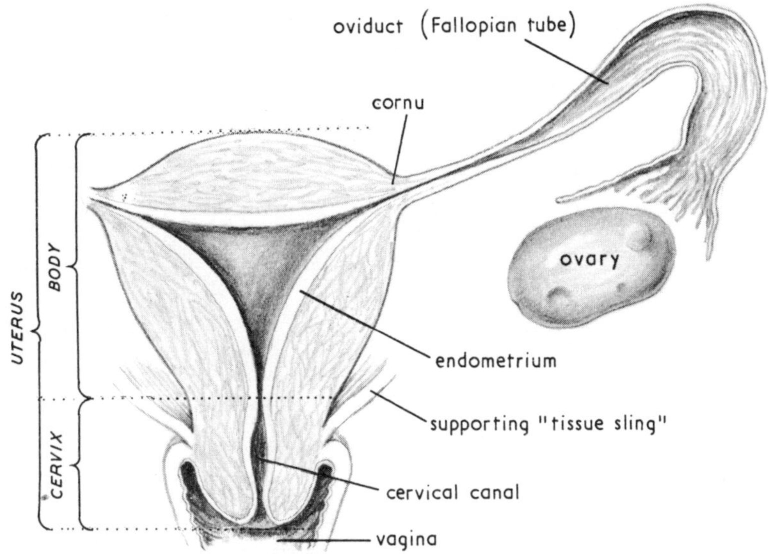

FIG. 1/5. The cavity of the uterus, and tubes

'prolapse' later in life. With better obstetrics, this complication is today much less likely to occur.

Normally the uterus lies bent forward at an angle of 90° to the vagina, resting on the bladder. As the bladder fills, it rotates backwards; as it empties, the uterus falls forward. In about 10 per cent of women the uterus lies bent backwards. This is called *retroversion*. In the past it was considered a serious condition, causing backache, sterility and many other complaints. There were many operations for its cure. Today it is known that unless the retroversion is due to infection or to a peculiar condition called endometriosis, it is unimportant and is not the cause of the symptoms which were attributed to it. Surgery is not needed, and the patient can be reassured that the position of the uterus is normal for her.

The *oviducts* (or Fallopian tubes) are two small, hollow tubes, one on each side, which stretch for about 10 cm. (4 in.) from the upper part of the uterus to lie in contact with the ovary on each side. The outer end of each oviduct is divided into long finger-like processes, and it is thought that these sweep up the egg when it is expelled from the ovary. The oviduct is lined with cells shaped like goblets, which lie between cells with frond-like borders. The oviduct is of great importance, as it is within it that fertilization of the egg takes place, and it is likely that its secretions help to nourish the fertilized egg as it is moved by the cells with long fronds towards the uterus.

The two *ovaries* are ovoid-shaped organs, averaging 3.5 cm. ($1\frac{1}{2}$ in.) in length and 2 cm. ($\frac{3}{4}$ in.) in breadth. In the infant they are small, delicate, thin structures, but after puberty they enlarge to reach the adult proportions mentioned. After the menopause, they become small and wrinkled, and in old age are less than half their adult size. Each ovary has a centre made up of small cells and a mesh of vessels. Surrounding this is the ovary proper–the cortex–which contains about 200,000 egg cells lying in a cellular bed (the stroma), and outside again, protecting the egg cells and the ovarian stroma, is a thickened layer of tissue. The ovaries are the equivalent of the male testes, and in addition to containing the egg cells on which all human life depends, are a hormone factory producing the female sex hormones, which are so important.

As can be appreciated, the passage within the genital tract extends from the vestibule, along the vagina, through the cervix and uterus, and along the tubes to the ovaries. It is because of this that the male spermatozoa can reach the female egg for fertilization to take place within the body.

CHAPTER 2

How human life begins

The human being, so complex in his behaviour, so different from his fellows, develops from a single fertilized cell. This cell–the fertilized ovum–divides almost at once into two identical cells. These two cells divide to make four identical cells, which then divide again, and so on. As they divide again and again, certain groups of cells become different, or differentiate, and form particular tissues or organs. For example, some cells form the bony skeleton, some the muscles, others the heart and blood vessels. Still others form the red blood cells which carry oxygen in the blood to the tissues, and others form the white blood cells which protect us against infections. Yet another group of cells multiplies to form the nerve cells of the brain and the nerves.

All these groups of cells with different functions have come from the single fertilized egg cell, and each and every cell has in its substance the information needed to perform the functions of any other cell, although once it has differentiated, it never does. Half of this information comes from the father's side of the family, and is transmitted in the spermatozoon which fertilized the egg. The other half comes from the mother's side, and is transmitted in the substance of the egg itself.

The information needed for the cell to perform its particular function is contained in the twisted strands of a substance found in the centre (or nucleus) of every cell. These strands are called chromosomes, and themselves are formed of long strings of several million beads, which are more properly called genes. The gene is the smallest unit of information, and is itself composed of twisted strands of a chemical called DNA (deoxyribonucleic acid). If you can imagine an ultra-sophisticated computer, which responds to requests fed in by giving out information, you have a pretty good idea of how the genes work in the cell. In any cell only a few genes operate to control the functions of that cell, the rest being covered over and inactive.

Each cell in the human body, with the exception of the egg cells in the woman and the spermatozoa in the man, contains 46 chromosomes. Forty-four of these chromosomes control all our physical characteristics and our body functions. These are called autosomes. The other two determine our sex. Recently it has been possible to take photographs of the chromosomes in the human body cells. In this way they can be displayed and measured. The two sex chromosomes can be identified easily. The smallest one has the shape of a Y, and is called the Y sex chromosome; the other has the shape of an X, and is called the X sex chromosome. Each of the millions of cells which make up a woman's body has 44 autosomes and two X chromosomes. A man's body cells have 44 autosomes, an X and a Y chromosome. You can see that even in the smallest body cell, a man is different from a woman because his cells alone have the Y chromosome.

As I have noted, the only cells in the body which do not have 46 chromosomes are the egg cells in the woman and the spermatozoa in the man. These two kinds of cells have only 23 chromosomes, and develop in special ways.

THE DEVELOPMENT OF THE EGG CELLS

Very early in life (about 20 days after fertilization) certain cells develop in the wall of the gut cavity of the embryo. These cells then migrate through the tissues to reach a thickened area lying in a ridge at each side of the midline of the gut cavity. This is the tissue from which the ovary will develop. By the 30th day after fertilization, the cells have settled in the tissue (which is now called a gonad), and have begun to multiply. By 140 days after fertilization (the 22nd week of pregnancy), a total of 7 million cells are found in the ovary, and many of them have acquired a coating of cells derived from the gonad. They develop within this protective coat, and fluid appears in many of the cells. These are the egg cells (or *oocytes*), and the cells which contain fluid are called *follicles*. The cells which do not have the coating are destroyed, and by birth only 2 million oocytes remain. In the childhood years, many of the oocytes are destroyed and by puberty only 200,000 remain. Each month from puberty to the menopause between 12 and 30 of the oocytes develop further, and one which outstrips all the rest in growth is expelled from the ovary. This is the ovum which may be fertilized. Occasionally more than one ovum escapes from the ovary. If the additional ova are fertilized twins, triplets or quadruplets will result, although twins may occur through another mechanism.

During its development in the ovary, the ovum divides into two daughter egg cells. This division is unequal, a large cell and a small cell being formed. Each of these cells has 23 chromosomes–22 autosomes and an X chromosome. The large cell is the one which will accept the head of the spermatozoon into its substance at the time of fertilization, and will form the new individual. The small cell is pushed to lie just inside the zona pellucida, and has no further function. It is called a *polar body*.

THE DEVELOPMENT OF THE SPERMATOZOA

It can be seen that all the egg cells in the ovary of the female are formed before birth, and none can be formed later. The male is different, spermatozoa are continually being formed in his testicles from puberty onwards, and into old age.

The spermatozoa are formed from parent cells found in the testicles. They undergo several changes before becoming mature, and during the changes the number of chromosomes in each spermatozoon is reduced by half. The mature spermatozoon therefore has 23 chromosomes. Twenty-two of these are autosomes and one is a sex chromosome. Since the parent sperm cell had 44 autosomes, an X and a Y chromosome, it follows that when it divides to form the spermatozoa, each will have 22 autosomes and an X *or* a Y chromosome (Fig. **2/1**). In this way two equal populations of spermatozoa form, and when you remember that each time a man has an orgasm he ejaculates between 100 and 400 *million* spermatozoa, they are large populations of cells. One population of spermatozoa has 22 autosomes and an X chromosome, the other 22 autosomes and a Y chromosome. If a spermatozoon carrying the Y chromosome fertilizes the egg, the new cell will have 44 autosomes, an X chromosome and a Y chromosome. The baby resulting from this will be a boy. If the spermatozoon which fertilizes the egg is one with 22 autosomes and an X chromo-

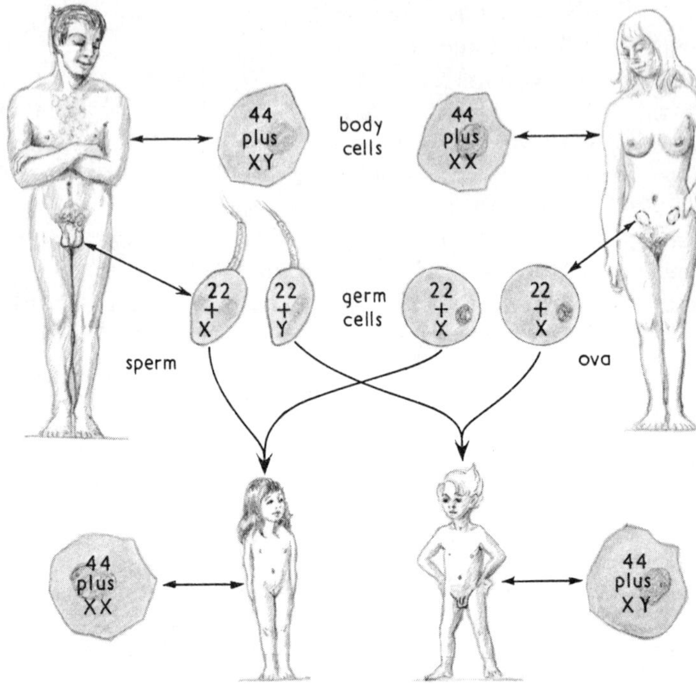

FIG. 2/1. The chromosomes of the ovum and spermatozoon

some, the resulting cell will have 44 autosomes and two X chromosomes. The baby resulting from this will be a girl (Fig. **2/1**). This means that the father determines the sex of the child.

THE FERTILIZATION OF THE EGG

A new life begins when a single spermatozoon, out of the millions which were deposited in the upper part of the vagina during intercourse, fertilizes the egg (or ovum). Of the millions of spermatozoa deposited in the vicinity of the cervix, only a few thousand manage to negotiate the twisting mucous tunnels of its canal to reach the cavity of the uterus. Of these only a few hundred get past the narrow part from the uterus to enter the oviduct, and only a few dozen swim up along the oviduct against the current made by the moving fronds of its lining to reach the ovum. Only one penetrates through the cells and tough, glistening, transparent 'shell' (the zona pellucida) which surrounds the egg. Once the spermatozoon has penetrated the 'shell' of the egg, it alters the zona pellucida in some way, so that no other spermatozoa are able to penetrate it. In this way only one spermatozoon fertilizes the ovum. The new life actually begins when the chromosomes of the ovum and those of the spermatozoon fuse together. Under the control of the genes, the cell then divides again and again until a human being is formed, as was described in the opening paragraph of this chapter.

The spermatozoon has a head, a middle-piece and a tail (Fig. **2/2**).

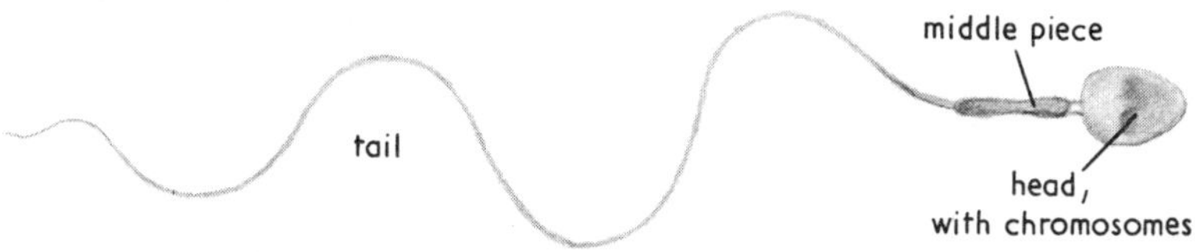

FIG. 2/2. The spermatozoon. The length is 0.05 mm. and the thickness of the tail is about half that of a fine hair. It is only visible under a microscope

The head contains the chromosomes, the middle-piece supplies the energy, and the tail propels it on its journey through the woman's genital tract (Fig. **2/3**). When the spermatozoon reaches the ovum, its head penetrates the outer shell, and enters the substance of the egg. The head then separates from the middle-piece and tail, which remain stuck in the shell and are destroyed.

When the head of the spermatozoon enters the ovum, its nucleus (which is the part containing the chromosomes) loses its wall and the chromosomes are exposed. Simultaneously, the wall surrounding the nucleus of the ovum is shed. The two sets of 23 chromosomes move together and fuse, so the number of chromosomes in the cell is 46 once again (Fig. **2/4**). In this way the number of chromosomes in the human body cell is kept constant at 46.

A woman is a woman because each cell in her body (with the exception of the egg cells) has 44 non-sex chromosomes and two X sex chromosomes. Her femininity is further confirmed by the fact that none of her body cells contains a Y chromosome. In the absence of a

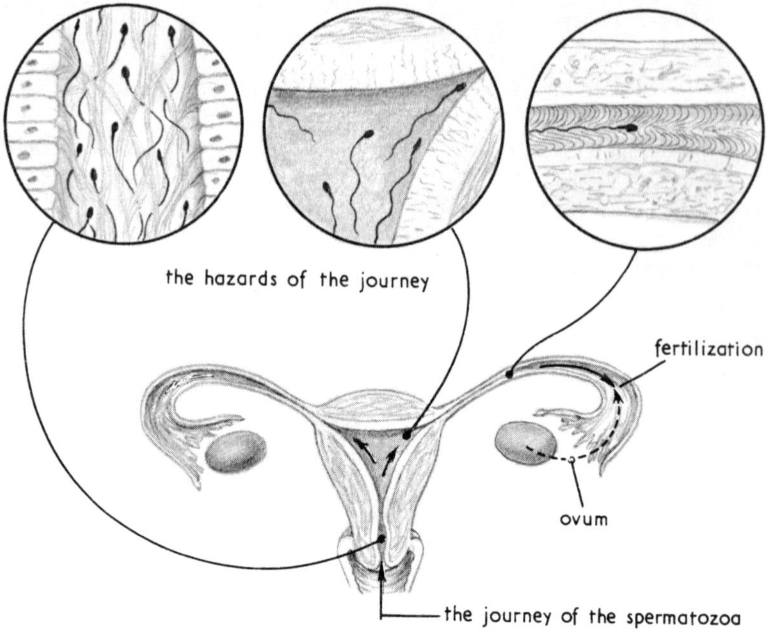

FIG. 2/3. The journey of the spermatozoa through the genital tract

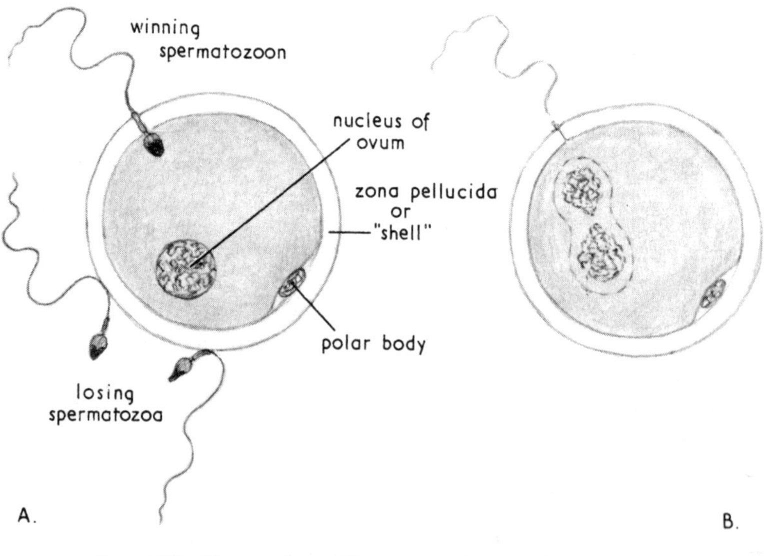

FIG. 2/4. Conception. The sperm head is seen in the substance of the egg in A, and the two exposed masses of genetic material are seen in B. Almost immediately they fuse and a new individual is formed

Y chromosome, her internal and external genitalia will develop in a feminine way. There is also some evidence that the absence of a Y chromosome tends to make her 'psychologically' feminine. The effect of this is small, however, compared with the very considerable psychological pressures during childhood which confirm her in her feminine role. She is treated from the time she can notice anything as a girl; she is shown to be different from boys; she performs different tasks; is expected to behave differently, and so rapidly realizes that she is female.

CHAPTER 3

The start of femininity

The moment that the newborn baby is breathing properly, the doctor examines it to make sure it is normal in every way, and hands it to the mother to fondle and cuddle. She has done something no man can do – she has matured a new life in her uterus for 40 weeks and her baby has been born.

The newborn baby is totally dependent on others for all its needs, and forms its first physical contact with its mother. If she is going to breast-feed the baby, its first real tactile contact is the soft, warm breast, which provides a pleasant food. Even if she does not breast-feed her baby, it is she who cuddles the infant, lavishes affection on it, and performs the many tasks needed to sustain its life. The emotional links between infant and its mother are strong, and a bond can also develop between infant and its father if he plays a proper role, sharing with his wife the care of the child. But the bond between infant and mother is so strong that the development of the growing child is influenced considerably by its character. If the mother is a warm, friendly person, the chances are that the child will develop in a similar way. If the mother is hard and unyielding, the child may reflect these characteristics, and find it difficult to adjust to a more normal human relationship in adult life. The sexual implications of this are no less important for the female than for the male.

The first sense an infant develops is touch, and although the warmth it obtains from cuddling is pleasurable, the infant soon begins to explore. The first explorations are necessarily confined to his own body, and the infant finds that touching the genital area produces pleasurable sensations. Similar pleasurable sensations are produced when the baby is bathed or the nappies (diapers) are changed. These explorations are completely normal.

As the infant grows and enters childhood, its sexual curiosity continues, and by the age of five it is curious about the opposite sex. Small children often play 'doctors'; the boy compares his anatomy with the girl. If parents treat sex as 'dirty', and threaten to punish a child found engaged in sexual play, the child may develop attitudes to sex which will mar his or her adult life.

THE FEMALE ROLE

Children of both sexes if left alone will occupy themselves in the same way, will play the same games and will see no difference (other than an anatomical one) between each other. However, few children are left in this natural state. From the moment the baby becomes a child, the parents reinforce the sexual difference between boys and girls, and emphasize their different roles. This sexual differentiation is also emphasized by the manufacturers of children's goods, finding its most ridiculous and extreme expression in the U.S.A. in the manufacture of 'bras' and cosmetics for children of 10 and 11. By all these influences, a gender role is established for each child, a role which is necessary for the survival of the nomadic tribe when man must hunt for meat and woman must cook, care for the children and occasionally grow vegetables. Moreover, the organizational pattern of tribal life demands that each sex knows its own duties and has its own responsibilities. Despite the television set, the car, the electric cooker, the water-heater and the suburban 'dream-home', we are in many ways as tribal as the natives of New Guinea or Equador. This tribalism may well be necessary – it certainly exists – and in its cultural atmosphere a girl is to a certain extent indoctrinated that her role is that of housewife and mother; one of her main objectives to get married and have children; her future to be encompassed by the walls of her 'dream-home'; her thoughts bounded by the family.

GYNAECOLOGICAL CONDITIONS IN CHILDHOOD

Since the genital organs are immature and have not been stimulated by the sex hormones which will be produced by the ovary at puberty, gynaecological problems in infancy are uncommon. However, two require mention, as they may cause distress.

The 'genital crisis'

A few female infants either bleed slightly from the vagina, or develop enlargement of the breasts which secrete a watery solution in the first week of life. These conditions are called the 'genital crisis', and are due to the passage from the mother to her baby of certain hormones. Following birth, the hormones no longer pass, and in a few infants the symptoms mentioned may occur. They are without significance; no treatment is required as they settle down and disappear within a few days.

Inflammation of the vulva and vagina

In small children the vulva and the vagina may become inflamed and sore. The inflammation may be due to irritation from soaps used for washing, to lack of washing and poor hygiene, which permit bacteria to grow, or to the introduction into the vagina of some object.

The condition is very painful, and medical help should be sought. Meanwhile, certain general principles of treatment can be adopted. These are: (1) general cleanliness, using only a mild soap, or none at all, for washing the child's vulva, (2) careful drying and powdering after vulval washing, and (3) the wearing of light, cotton panties day and night to prevent the child from scratching the area.

CHAPTER 4

Adolescence

The period of life between childhood and maturity is adolescence, which biologically extends from the age of 10 to the age of 19. The most important event in adolescence, as far as the girl and her mother are concerned, is the onset of menstruation, which may occur at any time between the ages of 10 and 16. The time of onset of menstruation is called the menarche. In rural societies the menarche was a mark that the girl was now a woman, and could take up the duties and obligations of womanhood. This cultural attitude is retained in many societies today. For some reason, which may be connected with better nutrition, the age of the onset of menstruation is becoming earlier. In Britain the average age of the onset of menstruation is now 13 years, compared with 15 years a century ago. It seems that the daughters of better-off parents tend to start menstruating a little earlier than those whose parents are poor, but the average difference is no more than 6 to 9 months. The old belief that the menarche occurred earlier in girls living in the hot tropics does not appear to be true, and the average age of onset of menstruation depends more on the socio-economic status of the parents than on the climate.

The menarche, however, is only the culminating change in a sequence which has altered the girl into a young woman. These changes are due to a series of interactions between several glands in the body. The controlling gland is a special part of the brain called the *hypothalamus*, which, working with the pituitary gland, controls the subsequent events. For reasons which are not yet clear, the hypothalamus begins to secrete substances called releasing factors about four years before the menarche. The releasing factors pass down the blood vessels connecting the hypothalamus to the pituitary, where they cause the release of several chemical substances, called hormones. One of these hormones is the growth hormone which causes the spurt of growth that precedes the menarche. The girl begins to grow about four years before the menarche, and the rate of growth is greatest in the first two years, slowing down as the menarche approaches.

Two other hormones secreted by the pituitary gland are of particular importance to women as they act on the egg cells in the ovaries. In Chapter 2 it was noted that by the time of birth, fluid had appeared in many of the egg cells, which were then called egg follicles. The first of the hormones which affects the egg cells is called the follicle-stimulating hormone (or FSH), because it stimulates the growth of some of the follicles. At first only a very few follicles grow, and as they do so their surrounding mantle of cells manufactures a hormone called oestrogen. This hormone is the one which makes a female child become a woman. The stimulated follicles produce oestrogen for about a month, and then die. But by this time other egg follicles have been stimulated, and these secrete oestrogen in their turn. As time passes, more follicles are stimulated each month (eventually between 12 and 20 being stimulated), so that there is a gradual rise in the amount of oestrogen produced by the ovaries. Oestrogen has many effects. It stimulates the growth of the ducts of the breasts and the area under the nipples, so that this becomes enlarged. It stimulates the growth of the oviducts, the uterus and the vagina. In the vagina it thickens the vaginal wall, and causes increased vaginal moisture. It causes fat to be laid down on the hips. It slows down the growth spurt which was started earlier by the pituitary growth hormone, so that the mature girl is generally not as tall as the mature boy.

As time passes, the amount of oestrogen in the circulation rises more rapidly, and the menarche is near. The rising levels of oestrogen stimulate the growth of the lining of the uterus (the *endometrium*), but at the same time 'feed-back' reduces the quantity of follicle-stimulating hormone secreted by the pituitary. Once the level of follicle-stimulating hormone begins to fall, the growth of the follicles in the ovaries and the secretion of oestrogen are reduced. The blood vessels supplying the lining of the uterus become kinked and break, so that bleeding occurs in the uterus. The endometrium crumbles. Blood and endometrial cells collect in the uterus, and then escape through the cervix into the vagina. Menstruation has started – the menarche has arrived.

The average age at which various changes occur is as follows:

Age 9–10	The bony pelvis begins to grow and to attain a female shape.
	Fat begins to be deposited, commencing the changes in shape to that of a woman.
	The nipples bud.
Age 10–11	The nipples increase in size.
	Hair begins to appear over the pubis.
Age 11–13	The area beneath the nipples develops.
	The internal and external genitals grow and develop.
	The vaginal wall thickens, and vaginal secretions may appear.
Age 12–14	The breasts develop further, and the nipples become darker in colour.
Age 13–15	Hair increases over the pubis, and appears in the arm-pits.
	Spots appear on the face of about half the girls.
	The menarche occurs, but the first few periods occur at irregular intervals.
Age 15–17	Increased fatty deposition occurs on the hips and the breasts.
	The periods become more regular.
Age 16–18	Growth of the skeleton ceases. The girl has now reached her maximum height.

MENSTRUATION

At intervals from the menarche–irregularly at first but with increasing regularity as time goes by–the girl 'has her periods', or menstruates. Within 4 to 6 years of the menarche (by the age of 17 to 19), her menstrual pattern will have become established. Each individual has her own pattern, but in most women menstruation occurs each month (unless pregnancy intervenes) until about the age of 45, when it becomes increasingly irregular once again. For convenience, the menstrual cycle is considered to start on the first day of menstruation (day 1), and to end the day before the next menstruation starts. The menstrual cycle therefore includes the days when bleeding occurs and the interval between each menstrual period. In most women the cycle varies in length from 24 to 34 days, averaging 29 days. But even the woman who says she knows exactly on what day menstruation will start is often a few days out either side. In adolescence, until the pattern has been established, menstruation tends to occur at irregular intervals, usually of longer duration than normal, but occasionally more frequently. In the first year or two after the menarche, the periods may only recur twice or three times a year, and when they do occur may be heavy. Sooner or later, however, a regular rhythmic pattern is established.

The menstrual cycle

It has been said that menstruation is 'the uterus weeping because pregnancy did not happen'. Bleeding from the crumbling of the lining of the uterus is the culmination of a series of interlocked events which prepare the uterus to accept a fertilized egg. If pregnancy does not occur, this prepared lining is shed from the uterus, and the whole cycle of events begins again.

The ultimate 'controller' of these events is the hypothalamus, and even this part of the brain is affected by emotions and upsets. This is demonstrated by the fact that menstruation may cease after a particularly strong emotional upset, or if a girl leaves home and changes her occupation. The duration of time during which menstruation ceases is variable and the periods usually return after two or three months; but in some patients the absence of the periods (which is called amenorrhoea) may last for more than a year. Such patients require careful investigation to exclude an underlying disease which may cause amenorrhoea. Luckily the cause is not usually a disease, and menstruation can be restored with certain drugs if this is considered desirable. It should be stressed that if there is no underlying disease, the absence of menstruation is of no importance. Contrary to a popular myth, menstruation does not clean the body, and the absence of menstruation does not mean that 'dangerous substances' are dammed up within the uterus.

As the sequence of events leading to each menstrual period is complicated, it is perhaps best to start at the time of menstruation and trace what happens up to the time of the next menstruation.

During menstruation the hypothalamus sends quantities of the FSH-releasing factor to stimulate the cells in the pituitary gland which manufactures FSH. The amount of FSH in the blood rises and stimulates a number of egg follicles in the ovary, usually 12 to

20. These follicles grow, and as they do so they manufacture oestrogen, so that the amount of this special female sex hormone increases in the blood. As has been noted earlier, oestrogen has several effects upon the tissues which make up the genital tract, but the one in which we are particularly interested is its action on the lining of the uterus. Oestrogen stimulates the lining to grow. At the end of menstruation most of the lining has crumbled away and, mixed with blood, has been shed as the menstrual flow. The lining is made up of narrow tubes, called endometrial glands, set in several layers of cells, called endometrial stomal cells. Oestrogen makes the glands grow, and the layers of stromal cells increase, or proliferate. Because of this, the changes in the uterus are called proliferative, and this part of the cycle is called the proliferative phase of the cycle.

As the follicles grow, the amount of oestrogen in the blood continues to rise, and by 13 days after the onset of menstruation, it has increased six-fold above the level found at its onset. The rising blood levels have an effect called a 'feed-back' on the hypothalamus, causing a reduction in FSH-releasing factor, but making the hypothalamus release another substance called the LH-releasing factor. This factor is carried down the blood vessels which connect the hypothalamus to the pituitary gland, where certain specialized cells produce a substance called luteinising hormone, or LH (Fig. **4/1**). This hormone is so-called because it induces one of the egg follicles to burst and expel its contained egg, and it then changes the cells which make up the follicle to a bright yellow colour. The Latin word for yellow is 'luteus'–hence the luteinising, or yellow-making hormone. At about the 14th day after the onset of menstruation (in a girl with a normal cycle, or later if the cycle is prolonged unduly) a sudden surge of luteinising hormone sweeps through the blood stream. It reaches the ovary, where it induces 'bursting' of the egg follicle which has grown the most, and which is blown-up and tight like a tiny balloon. During growth, this particular follicle has swollen and moved through the ovary to reach its surface, where it makes a tiny bulge that can be seen by the naked eye. Suddenly, under the influence of the luteinising hormone, the follicle bursts and the egg is pushed out, together with the fluid in which it lay. The egg is caught in the finger-like ends of the oviduct which caress the ovary at this time, and is moved slowly but gently into the cavity of the oviduct tube, where fertilization takes place, if this is to happen (Fig. **4/2**).

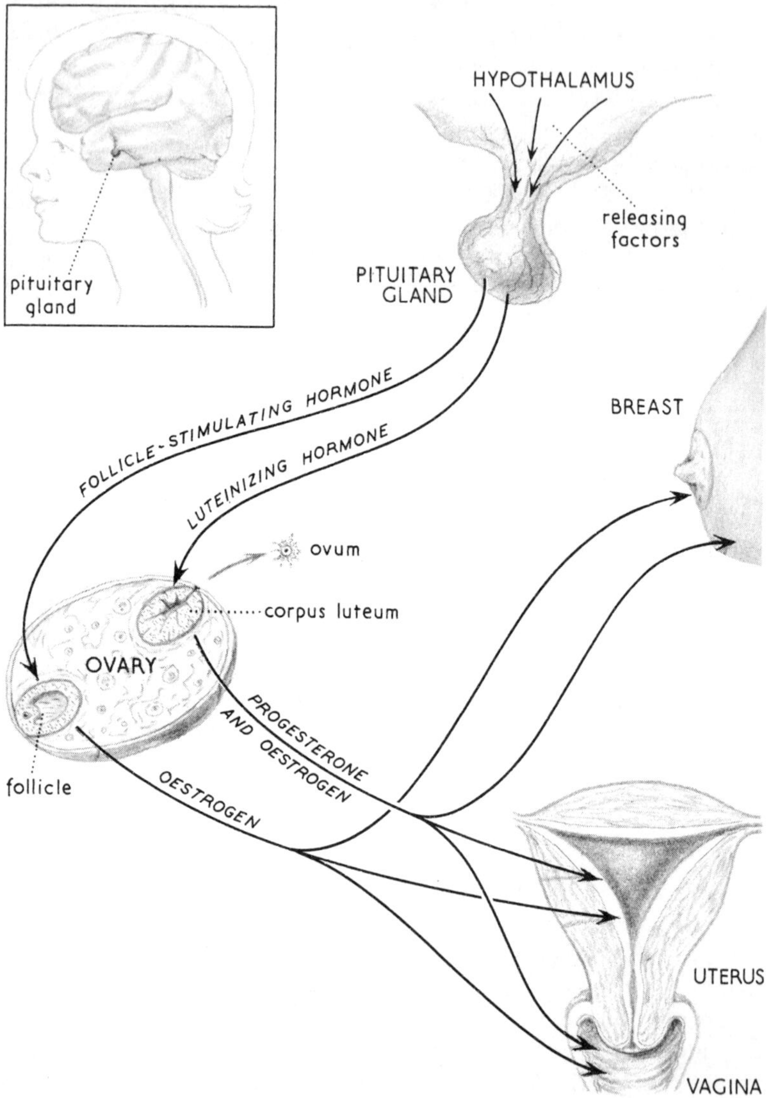

FIG. 4/1. The control of menstruation

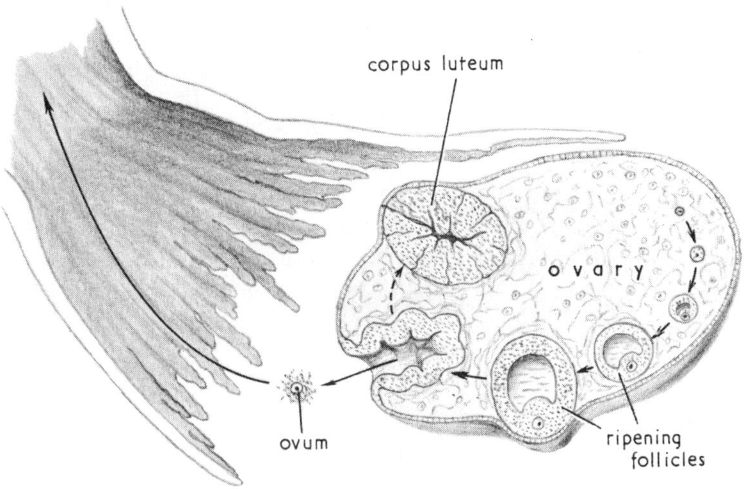

FIG. 4/2. The growth of stimulated follicles in the ovary during a menstrual cycle

Once the egg (or ovum) has been expelled, the now-empty follicle collapses, and the luteinising hormone acts on the cells of its wall, turning them yellow. The collapsed follicle is called a yellow body, or, in Latin, a *corpus luteum*. The change in colour of the cells of the corpus luteum is due to a change in their activity. Now not only do they continue to secrete oestrogen (along with the other 11 to 19 stimulated follicles which failed to grow so quickly), but uniquely they also manufacture a new hormone called progesterone. The name is apt, for the hormone prepares the uterus for pregnancy (*pro-gestos*)–hence pro-gest-erone (*-one* indicates the kind of chemical substance). Progesterone is the second main female sex hormone. It has many actions, but the main ones are that it relaxes smooth (involuntary) muscle; increases the production of the waxy secretions of the skin; and raises the temperature of the body. This is why it is normal for women in the second half of the menstrual cycle to have a temperature up to 37.4° Centigrade, or 99.5° Fahrenheit. The most important progestational effect of progesterone is its action on the uterus. Progesterone thickens the lining of the uterus, and induces the glands to secrete a nutritious fluid and become succulent, so that the fertilized egg may be nourished during the time it needs to take root or implant in the lining of the womb. The part of the menstrual cycle after ovulation is called the secretory or progestational phase.

Unless the egg is fertilized and implants onto the endometrium, the yellow body in the ovary dies (as do the other stimulated follicles). If this happens, the level of oestrogen and progesterone in the blood falls. This has two effects: firstly, the restraint on FSH-releasing factors by the hypothalamus is removed, and FSH production by the pituitary gland increases. Secondly, without the stimulation of oestrogen and progesterone, the now thick, juicy lining of the uterus begins to shrink, and in doing so kinks the tiny blood vessels which supply it. The kinked blood vessels (really blood capillaries) break, and patchy bleeding occurs in the deeper layers of the lining. This separates the lining above the blood; it crumbles and is shed into the uterine cavity, together with blood. Within a few hours, the amount of blood in the uterine cavity is such that the uterus contracts, expelling the blood through the cervix into the vagina. Menstruation has begun.

'Protection' in menstruation

No woman wants to discolour her clothes with menstrual blood. In the past a rag was used which was placed over the vulva, and which is the origin of an English name for menstruation – 'the rags'. Today clean, absorbent, easily-disposable materials are used to make sanitary pads and intravaginal tampons, the two usual ways of dealing with menstrual loss. The sanitary pad has the disadvantage that it may chafe the upper thighs as it lies applied to the vulva, and may be apparent, particularly in sports clothes. The latter objection is often more in the mind of the wearer than of the observer, and if menstruation is considered a normal function (which it is), it is surely unimportant if others know that a menstrual period is in progress. It is only in communities which consider menstruation something of which to be ashamed and to be hidden that these attitudes apply.

The intravaginal tampon has the advantage that it is convenient, inconspicuous and effective. There is no truth in the belief that it is dangerous to collect menstrual blood in the vagina. Since the tampon must be introduced into the vagina, it should not be used in the early years of puberty, but by the age of 16 or 17 it may replace the sanitary pad, provided the girl can introduce it without discomfort. A disadvantage is that occasionally a tampon may be forgotten and left in the vagina. This can lead to a most offensive vaginal discharge. Women who have profuse periods also find that the tampon is inadequate to mop up the blood loss, and may find a sanitary pad more satisfactory. The choice is that of the girl–neither method is superior to the other, both being satisfactory.

Myths about menstruation

In primitive cultures, menstruating women were regarded not as dirty, but as evil and dangerous. The loss of blood to primitive races was a loss of life. As menstrual blood emerged from the same passage as did the baby, but seemed in some way to prevent pregnancy, it was felt to be a danger to growing things. A menstruating woman therefore could damage crops, cause animals to abort, turn wine into vinegar and turn milk sour by her presence. These primitive beliefs are still accepted in parts of Europe today, and it is believed that if a menstruating woman makes jam it will not keep; if she touches wine, beer or milk it will go bad; if she touches buds they will wither; and if she rides a pregnant mare it will miscarry. In most societies it was therefore felt imperative that a woman, at the time of the menstrual period, withdrew from the life of the community, and remained secluded and hidden from view in the house. Whilst menstruating, she could not touch food or cook, nor should her shadow fall on another woman, particularly if she was pregnant. These strange prohibitions are found in Australian Aboriginal tribes, and amongst the highly intelligent but superstitious Hindu cultures. Almost all societies have surrounded menstruation with myth and ritual. Both the Jews and the Muslims have elaborate rituals for purification following menstruation, and even in modern Western society strange traditional beliefs persist. Certain foods, especially pineapple and raspberries, are thought to be 'bad' if eaten during menstruation. Washing the hair is believed to lead to an increased menstrual loss, and to the development of a cold or pneumonia.

Of course, there is no basis of truth in any of these beliefs. Provided the menstrual flow is not too heavy and the girl wishes, she can take part in any activity. She can ride, swim, work or walk, wash her head or her feet, eat what she likes, bathe or shower, dance or drive.

Menstrual irregularities in adolescence

The menstrual cycle is repeated throughout the reproductive years, unless pregnancy occurs. At each extreme – that is in adolescence and near the menopause – the cycles are less regular, and ovulation may not occur. In these cycles the endometrium is only stimulated by oestrogen, and only FSH is secreted (in any quantity) by the pituitary gland. The menstrual cycles tend to be irregular in duration: they may be as short as 12 days, or as long as 3 or 4 months. The duration and amount of menstrual bleeding is also variable: it may be scanty and of short duration, or heavy and long. If the bleeding times are too heavy or too prolonged, the girl should consult a doctor who can give hormonal treatment for a few months to regulate the periods. During this time, the girl's own rhythm is established. In most cases, the irregularity is not too inconvenient, and the knowledge that normal cycles will eventually appear is sufficient reassurance. But if there is any doubt, the girl should consult a doctor.

DELAYED ONSET OF MENSTRUATION

Of even more concern to the girl, and more particularly to her mother, is when the periods fail to start. If menstruation has not started by the age of 16, and particularly if the girl is of short stature, a doctor should be consulted. He will take a very careful history, will require to make a full physical examination, and finally will need to make a pelvic examination (although in some cases an examination by inserting a finger into the rectum will give sufficient information). If at the end of this time the doctor has not been able to find out why the periods have not started, the girl should be referred to a gynaecologist so that special investigations can be started. The investigations are fairly simple and include the examination under a microscope of cells taken by a swab from the inside of the cheek. Other tests are to estimate the amount of female sex hormones in a specimen of urine collected over a 24-hour period, and possibly more complex investigations to find the chromosome pattern of the body cells.

DYSMENORRHOEA

Many girls suffer from painful periods. This is called dysmenorrhoea. Dysmenorrhoea does not usually start until two or three years after the menarche, and usually only occurs if the menstrual period follows a cycle in which ovulation occurred. Occasionally dysmenorrhoea occurs in a period in which ovulation did not occur (called an 'anovulatory cycle'), particularly if the menstrual blood clots in the uterus, and the small clots are then expelled.

The pain is cramp-like in character, felt in the lower abdomen, and usually starts 24 hours before the menstrual period and lasts for the first 12 hours of bleeding, when all the discomfort goes.

The cause of dysmenorrhoea is unknown, but the most acceptable theory is that the pain is caused by spasm of the uterine muscle, due in turn to an immature blood supply. The cause of the pain is therefore similar to that which occurs in your arm if you tie a tight band around the upper part. Cultural beliefs, and the concept that menstruation is the discharge of waste products, have the effect of increasing the pain sensation. Thus adolescents in 'primitive races' are said to suffer less dysmenorrhoea than girls in more sophisticated Western societies. It is by no means certain that this is true, but Western society in calling menstruation 'the curse', the 'poorly time' and the 'unclean time' (as in the Bible) only intensifies the erroneous belief that menstruation is something of which to be ashamed, and not the naturally-occurring shedding of the uterine lining prepared for a pregnancy which failed to occur.

Probably 50 per cent of women complain of dysmenorrhoea at some stage of their life. Usually the peak years are between 17 and 25, and the condition is relieved or cured by pregnancy. Because of this high incidence, a bewildering variety of treatments have been prescribed in the past, and continue to appear today. Some of the more bizarre methods, such as exotic spinal and pelvic exercises, Sitz baths, cold showers, and surgical operations for removing the nerves of the pelvis, are now of only historical interest, but others equally wild appear from time to time.

The great majority of girls need no more than an explanation of what dysmenorrhoea is, a sympathetic attitude from parents which is neither too hard nor too pitying, and the use of aspirin or other pain-killing drugs. If the pain is so incapacitating that the girl has to go to bed, or has associated vomiting, the use of the oral contraceptives ('the Pill') will usually prevent dysmenorrhoea. Another hormonal treatment, which prevents dysmenorrhoea apparently without stopping ovulation, has been introduced recently. Although effective, neither of these treatments should be used until the girl has been examined by a doctor.

EMOTIONAL CHANGES IN ADOLESCENCE

The tremendous changes in the girl's body which occur during puberty are matched by psychological and emotional changes. During these years each facet of the girl's growth and development affects other facets, and her task of adjustment can be helped or hindered by parental attitudes. At this time she begins to feel the force of new, ill-understood heterosexual attractions. It is the time of hero-worship and devotion to a succession of teenage idols. It is a time of emotional storms and a feeling of not being understood. It is a time when previously accepted beliefs are questioned. It is a time when the tides of hormonal changes are matched by tides of emotional uncertainty. The young teenager needs sympathetic understanding. She needs to be treated as a young adult, and not as an overgrown infant. Her questions regarding social, moral and sexual attitudes must be answered with this in mind. If parents are unable to do this, they hamper their child's period of adjustment.

CHAPTER 5

Sex in the life of a woman

In these days of change – social, educational and sexual – the obvious differences between man and woman have been reduced considerably. Although a woman tends to have less well-developed muscles than a man, she equals him in physical and mental stamina, and is able increasingly to perform jobs which have been reserved for men in the past. The degree to which this change has occurred varies between countries, but more and more the two sexes are performing the same work and are sharing responsibilities previously reserved for one or the other. Political power, industrial power and military power – the three props which support Western society at present – are still predominantly male preserves, but even here increasing numbers of women are playing a significant part and sharing power with men. Biologically, woman is unique as she alone is needed for the survival of the race. One man can sire many children, but each child needs to grow within a woman's uterus, to be born at a specific time, and to be nurtured in childhood by its mother.

In the earliest tribal societies, the whole culture was predominantly feminine, centring round child-rearing, food-getting and home-making. The women tilled such fields as there were, and cultivated the edible vegetables. Man had far less responsibility. He brought in food from hunting, he took part in certain rituals necessary to bring rain or deflect the anger of the gods, he occasionally helped with certain limited duties. Once nomadic tribes settled, cultivated fixed fields and domesticated animals, man began to dominate society. His status in his tribe could be measured by the number of his cattle or goats, and women became debased to be possessions of man, ranking only a bit above his cows. In the West, by the Middle

Ages women of the peasant class had lost all of their traditionally dominant duties, and now worked in the fields and in the house under the guidance and dominance of the man, who considered woman his chattel. If a woman was born into the upper classes, she did little except grace the house, organize the servants and act chiefly as a toy or pet for her husband. In India, Hindu society had strict rules for the conduct of the sexes, which hardly changed over 2,000 years. The woman entered her husband's family at marriage and the primary object of marriage was the birth of a son so that the family line might continue. The woman was therefore totally subordinate to her husband, who believed that she was inferior to man, less able to resist temptation and therefore weaker. Because of this, it was his duty to protect his wife with 'the respect due to his mother', but also to regulate her behaviour to his desires.

The early Christian cultures of the West also held that woman was inferior to man, and following St. Augustine believed that sexual intercourse was evil and really only permissible for the purpose of producing children, a belief similar to that of the older Hindu religion. The pronouncements of the early Christian theologians were further codified during the turbulence of the Reformation, when male dominance and female subjugation were confirmed. This strengthened the 'double standard' of sexual behaviour–which had existed before the Reformation and is still apparent today. The double standard permits the male to seek sexual satisfaction with women, and even encourages him to do so, whilst the female is expected to remain a virgin until marriage and then submit to male dominance.

Escape from this rigid pattern of male dominance and female submission only came after the investigations of Sigmund Freud towards the end of the nineteenth century had shown that sex was a basic instinct, which might be enjoyed by both men and women. Other psychological investigators amplified Freud's original work by confirming that sex should extend beyond the mere physical act of copulation to involve the emotional responses of both partners. In other words, the knowledge and involvement of both partners in sex was needed for the further development of their personalities in marriage. The more permissive attitude to sexual matters which has occurred in recent years in Western society derives from these original findings. It has been encouraged by the emancipation of woman from the bondage of the home.

This does not necessarily mean a reduction in the degree of femininity of woman. All mammals, including man, have patterns of behaviour in which one sex displays its charms to attract the other for sexual purposes. In human females this is evident, and the adolescent and young adult girl in every culture–whether Western or Eastern–has these feminine attributes, but in each culture she is taught certain controls, and learns acceptable ways of expressing her femininity. In the West in the Victorian era, for example, woman was demure and shy, and provocatively showed her ankle. In the late 1930s she was forthright and flaunted her breasts. Today she joins in with the male in many activities, their emotional and physical life is shared much more, but still she dresses to attract male eyes.

Nor does feminine emancipation from male dominance mean a reduction of the quality of a woman's home-building functions. The woman can manage her home, can rear her children and can still exercise her brain, whilst doing so. Once the children are independent, she can expand her interests beyond the home to encompass other activities and lead a fuller, more satisfying life. Many men are still antagonistic to this, perhaps feeling a threat to their masculinity, but their numbers are becoming fewer.

From this it can be seen that femininity is the result of a combination of physical and cultural factors, and includes a willingness to be a mother and a capacity to be sexually attractive to a man. This capacity does not necessarily mean that a woman is beautiful, for standards of beauty constantly change. For example, the 'pin-up' girl of the war years is singularly unattractive to the youth of today; she looks blowsy, blown-up and bleached. The capacity to be sexually attractive is deeper, and originates in qualities of character and behaviour, and can be found in women who are considered plain. Beauty which approximates to the current conventions gives the girl an additional advantage, but does not replace the qualities of character.

Having attracted the male, the femininity of the woman shows itself in her behaviour during sexual intercourse. Biologically woman is not as continuously receptive to or desirous of sexual intercourse as is the male. But she does not necessarily have to play an active part, beyond permitting coitus to take place, although today she is usually much more involved than that. The older values of female submission and lack of enjoyment of sexual intercourse are being replaced by a modern, more enlightened view that the woman should participate. This may put an additional strain on the male. Whereas in the older culture all he had to do was to achieve and maintain an erection, and reach an orgasm at his desired pace, now he is expected to help his wife achieve release from sexual tension if this is present. If woman is considered neither inferior nor submissive, but as a partner in marriage and a person whose sexual characteristics and behaviour are complementary to her husband's (as his are to hers), then the quality of her femininity is increased, and she and her husband can lead a fuller life.

Despite today's more rational attitude to sex, the collected myths of the last centuries still affect women, and can cause anxiety, unhappiness and concern. In this chapter, some of the old myths are examined and exposed as the nonsense they are, whilst other sexual problems are discussed in the hope that by reading about them, the problem may be resolved.

THE SEXUAL DRIVE

Just as different people have different appetites for food, for drink and for other sensual pleasures, individuals have different degrees of sexual drive, or need. The relative influence of genetic, instinctive and environmental factors on the sexual drive has not been fully elucidated. It is probable that individuals differ in the strength of their inherited sexual drive, but undoubtedly the environmental influences occurring during childhood and adolescence play a major part in determining the individual's adult sexual drive. In the case of a girl, the attitude of her parents towards sex, and especially that of her mother, seems important, although this can be modified by the attitudes of friends of her age group. A mother, for example, who brings up her daughter to believe that sex is evil, and that it is the duty of a wife to submit to, but not enjoy, sexual intercourse, may produce a girl whose sexual drive is markedly reduced. Similarly, parents whose attitude to sexual matters is so strict that they refuse to answer a child's natural questions about its origin, and about other sexual matters, and who condemn or punish the child for touching its genitals, are likely to warp its sexuality.

At the time of puberty, the hormonal secretions of the ovary initiate an interest in sexual matters, which has been latent since birth, but the strength of the interest (which is another way of saying the sexual drive) is conditioned by psychological influences which have occurred prior to puberty. These influences remain the key to the drive, but influences occurring during life can affect the sexual drive considerably, and it is known that it waxes and wanes throughout life without any recognizable pattern.

Although humans–both male and female–differ markedly in the amount of their sexual drive, conflict will only occur if a partner whose sexual drive is high marries one whose sexual drive is low. In other words, the relative sexual drive between the partners is of much more importance to their happiness than the absolute drive of each individual. A person is only 'oversexed' or 'undersexed' when compared with a specific sexual partner. The sexual drive is strongest in late adolescence and the early twenties, diminishing to a variable degree as the person gets older, particularly amongst men. The sexual drive of the female does not show this decline to such a degree. However, this is a gross generalization, and *individual* patterns are quite variable. Within the marriage, the degree of sexual drive of the wife seems to be more important than that of her husband in maintaining harmonious sexual relationships. This means that sexual harmony is obtained more easily if the wife's sexual drive equals or exceeds that of her husband. Problems arise more frequently if his drive is high, whilst hers is low. Either he suppresses his sexual drive, sublimating it in other occupations, or he releases it by taking an extramarital partner. If the wife's drive greatly exceeds her husband's, she finds it more difficult in the conditions of today's society to find an alternative partner, but seems to be more easily able to sublimate her urge in other ways. The relief may be obtained by involving herself in her home and children, or by taking up a job. Unfortunately her sexual frustration is often expressed in a variety of 'gynaecological' disorders, such as pain in the lower abdomen, backache, increased vaginal discharge, or changes in the character of her periods. In these conditions, the disorder lies in the mind, not the pelvis where it is manifested. These conditions are psychosomatic in origin, and are considered further in Chapter 19.

MASTURBATION

Stimulation of the genitalia by the fingers is almost universal in childhood, and in adolescence masturbation is general. Studies in several countries have shown that almost all young males masturbate, and three-quarters of females have masturbated by the age of 21. The frequency varies very considerably, but is higher amongst males. As the person gets older and heterosexual contacts are more readily available, the frequency of masturbation diminishes, although it continues throughout life. One way in which married couples obtain sexual contentment is by mutual masturbation, the male caressing his wife's clitoris and vulva, whilst she simultaneously strokes his penis. Masturbation is a normal part of sexual development, and does no harm whatsoever, however frequently or infrequently it takes place. The only problems which may result from it are feelings of guilt, occasioned by the Judao-Christian religious disapproval of masturbation. The young woman or man need have no feelings of guilt, since masturbation causes no bodily damage.

Strange, nonsensical myths are still perpetuated: masturbation is said to make a person weak, to damage his eyesight and, in excess (whatever that is), to cause brain decay or insanity. Masturbation does none of these things, but these particularly vicious ideas are still spread by ignorant people. In the female, masturbation has been said to lead to enlargement of the inner lips of the vulva, to 'congestion of the pelvis', and to venereal disease. Again, all these ideas are nonsensical.

At a higher level, masturbation has been declared as evidence of immaturity, which is clearly nonsense as people who are sexually well-adapted and mature find sexual contentment by masturbation, as well as by the more usual coital methods. It has been said that it leads to sexual frustration and frigidity, but as other equally distinguished investigators declare it leads to sexual excess, it is obvious that these objections are emotional not factual. It has been said that 'one cannot possibly get full emotional gratification through masturbation'. Whilst it is true that the greatest emotional gratification is obtained by giving to and receiving from a loved one, it is unfair to say that in masturbation something is lacking. In the absence of the loved one, masturbation whilst thinking of the loved one, or by making fantasies of other sexual situations, can lead to great emotional gratification. Of course, the truth is that masturbation is not harmful–no more in adult life than at any other time of life.

PETTING

Petting is the American term for love-making which reaches to, but stops short of, coitus. In other countries and at other times, other terms have been used: bundling, lolligagging, mugging, smooching. The activity is as old as tribal society, and is practised by tribes as primitive as those of New Guinea, or by people with cultures as sophisticated as that of the U.S.A. In Western countries, petting seems to be confined largely to adolescents. In 'light petting' (or 'necking'), the couple kiss passionately, their bodies (usually fully clothed) are in contact, but certain zones are 'forbidden' by the girl, who may refuse to allow her breasts to be caressed, and will not allow wandering hands to reach for her vulva. In 'heavy petting', passionate kissing, breast stimulation, caressing of the clitoris to orgasm, and of the penis to ejaculation, are accepted in varying degrees; but the girl remains a technical virgin as she does not allow the man's penis to enter her vagina.

Western society appears to accept petting, at least light petting, but to condemn pre-marital coitus. In doing so, it imposes restraints on the couple which are difficult to hold, and are often broken. Yet society in condemning coitus does have reason. Premarital coitus may lead to the transmission of syphilis or gonorrhoea from one infected partner to the other non-infected one, and it may lead to pregnancy. Since the sexual urges aroused by heavy petting may not be able to be withstood and copulation may result – as it often does – society's condemnation has a further danger: the girl may be ignorant of, or have not availed herself of, contraceptive measures so that pregnancy results.

The acceptance of petting as a social way of meeting sexual tensions may well arise from the nature of Western society: marriage often has to be delayed for economic reasons; the cold climate and urbanization reduces the opportunity for secluded love-making in the country; and the smallness of houses inhibits more intense love-making in the home, particularly with parents in a nearby room. Finally, there is the general availability of the car. The back seat is hardly the most romantic place, yet it may be the only place where the couple can obtain privacy, contact and warmth. Sexual intercourse in an automobile is of necessity brief, mechanical and uncomfortable, but 'heavy petting' in such a situation may relieve sexual tension without the unaesthetic associations of copulation in a car.

In present Western society petting appears to have a place in sexual development, but it may decline in popularity as more people accept that premarital intercourse is not only frequent (only 55 per cent of girls are virgin at the age of 20*), and provided it is not promiscuous, is a necessary sexual outlet in certain circumstances.

PREMARITAL SEXUAL INTERCOURSE

It is quite clear from investigation made in most Western countries that premarital sexual intercourse is not uncommon. Indeed, most cultures have been more lenient than ours in permitting premarital coitus, although all societies have imposed some sexual restraints to regulate it. In our society a double standard of sexual morality still exists to some extent. Premarital sexual intercourse is condemned both for males and females; but whilst the condemnation for girls is marked, society shows tolerance towards, or even a mild encouragement of, males who indulge in premarital coitus. In recent years a change of attitude has occurred, and a more permissive sexual atmosphere has arisen, particularly in Scandinavian countries, without a deterioration in moral standards.

In Australia, Britain and the U.S.A. where attitudes towards sex, and particularly premarital sexual intercourse, are sometimes less flexible, studies by responsible investigators have shown that more than 6 women in every 10 have had sexual intercourse before marriage, although in half of them coitus took place only with one partner, the fiancé or boy-friend. From this it is clear that sexual permissiveness is not the same thing as sexual promiscuity, in which the girl copulates with several partners, and no emotional bond is established with any of them. The promiscuous girl is emotionally insecure, and seeks security, status or notoriety by means of sex. Psychiatrists note a difference between females and males to premarital sexual expression, whether petting or sexual intercourse. Girls see premarital sex as a romantic expression of being in love,

*This figure comes from the following sources: the *Sunday Times* Survey 1970, a survey published in the *Medical Journal of Australia*, Kinsey's American report and Reiss's report in the *American Sociological Review*, **29**, 688.

whilst boys see sexual intercourse as a means of sexual relief, a status symbol amongst their group and a proof of their manhood.

However, it is clear that an increasing proportion of girls do have sexual intercourse before marriage, usually with their fiancé, and do not feel guilty about it. The deterrents that kept a girl a virgin before marriage are losing their impact. Opportunities for sexual intercourse are greater, because of the car and the bottle-party; the fear of venereal disease seems to have diminished, and the fear of pregnancy and disgrace is less strong. If the girl is promiscuous, or if her partner has been promiscuous, venereal disease is still a grave danger, particularly now that resistant germs have appeared, which require high doses of antibiotics and complex treatments for cure. But it seems that venereal disease is not a marked deterrent.

Pregnancy is an even greater hazard, and one of considerable consequence to the girl, to her family and to the community, particularly amongst young unmarried teenagers. This is of importance as the average age when a girl first has sexual intercourse appears to be between 17 and 19, and the average time between the first coitus and marriage is more than one year. Premarital pregnancies occur frequently. In Australia, for example, 8 per cent of all births are to unmarried mothers, and at least another 20 per cent of women conceive before marriage. Amongst the latter group, pregnancy is either terminated by an 'illegal' abortion or the marriage hastened, both potentially undesirable events. Information from Britain and the U.S.A. indicates that a similar proportion of premarital conceptions occur in those countries.

It seems of little avail for moralists and churchmen to appeal for a return to a stricter 'morality', particularly when the mass media, newspapers, magazines, cinema, radio and television emphasize sex. The old folk myth that premarital sexual intercourse, or unchastity of the female led to unhappiness, conflict and failure in marriage has been found to be untrue. Nor is there any evidence to suggest that widespread sex education will necessarily decrease the frequency of premarital sexual intercourse, although it should limit its consequences, and reduce promiscuity.

The answer seems to be that women will have to use their own pressure on society to create an environment in which it is possible for them to choose either to avoid sexual intercourse before marriage or to have premarital sexual intercourse, protected against the consequence of venereal disease by not being promiscuous, and against the risk of pregnancy by using a contraceptive. It is not enough that the boy says he 'will be careful', or will 'withdraw', or is 'prepared'. The girl must protect herself against pregnancy. In a study in Australia of 200 pregnant women, 70 per cent had had premarital intercourse, and 4 out of every 5 had left the contraception to the male, the result having been pregnancy.

The girl herself needs to take contraceptive measures, particularly as a change in sexual morality towards what might be called 'permissiveness with affection' is apparent. This means that premarital sexual intercourse when the girl is in love is being increasingly accepted. A hastened marriage and a child may create such stresses that the relations between the couple may be damaged irreparably, or the girl may decide to bear the child and have it adopted, a procedure which is very stressful and followed by a period of grief. Pregnancy can be prevented by adequate contraceptive measures. The choice lies between oral contraceptives ('the Pill'), the vaginal diaphragm (and spermicidal jelly), or the intrauterine contraceptive device (the Loop). Which is chosen depends on many, fairly complex factors, and for a choice to be made the girl must be able to obtain expert advice and full discussion, either from a 'family doctor' or at a family planning clinic, without feeling shame or guilt at her action.

APHRODISIACS

Since the dawn of time, erotic stimulants have been given to men who felt that their sexual performance was waning, and to women who failed to respond to sexual advances. The oldest existing medical textbook, an undated Egyptian scroll from about 2,000 B.C., contains recipes for making 'erotic potions'. More recently Shakespeare wrote extensively of aphrodisiacs. The great number of substances recommended as sexual stimulants indicates that none is of much value. Oysters are said to lead to amorous behaviour; rhinoceros horn powdered and drunk in wine is said to restore waning sexual function; whilst yohimbine, derived from the bark of an African tree, has long been used by the natives to increase their sexual powers. Cantharides, or Spanish fly, which is in fact an irritant of the urinary tract, also has an aphrodisiacal reputation. All these beliefs are baseless, and none of the many foods, drugs or irritants recommended through the ages has any aphrodisiacal property. Set apart, because of its frequent consumption in Western society, is alcohol. Alcohol, particularly champagne, is credited as being a considerable erotic stimulant. Alcohol, it is true, causes dilation of the skin blood vessels and a feeling of warmth which extends to the genitals. In small quantities it acts as a narcotic of the higher centres, producing a light-hearted approach and reducing the 'moral' block to sexual behaviour, but in larger quantities, its narcotic effect reduces rather than stimulates sexual desires and performance, as the Porter in *Macbeth* well knew:

'And drink, sir, is a great provoker of three things . . . Nose painting, sleep, and urine. Lechery, sir, it provokes and unprovokes; it provokes the desire, but it takes away the performance. Therefore much drink may be said to be an equivocator with lechery; it makes him and it mars him; it sets him on and it takes him off; it persuades him, and disheartens him; it makes him stand to, and not to stand to; in conclusion, equivocates him in a sleep, and, giving him the lie, leaves him.'

In summary, there is no such thing as a true aphrodisiac, and the drug that the eager male could induce the resistant female to take, which would render her unresisting and so full of sexual ardour that she would welcome seduction, does not exist. However, it must be admitted that the feelings of a woman for an escort who has given her a deliciously cooked meal, a reasonable quantity of good wine, in an intimate, well-furnished, candle-lit restaurant, are likely to be more amorous than if he had offered her a meatpie and potato chips in a brightly-lit café. But if she has no feeling towards him, the food and wine are not likely to change her opinion.

THE SEXUAL BACKGROUND TO MARRIAGE

A music-hall song goes, 'If women like that like men like those, why won't women like me?' That, in fact, just about sums up our knowledge of why, in our society, two people 'fall in love and marry'. In many societies, love is not a factor in marriage. In India, for example, marriages are often arranged by the family, who selects a suitable girl from one of several villages which traditionally supply brides to the village of the groom. The groom does not see his bride before the marriage. The evidence is that these marriages work fairly well; each partner knowing his or her duties and responsibilities, and the sexual aspect being limited. But in our society, the decision is made by the man and the woman that they will live together, will procreate and bring up children, will support each other, and will merge their personalities to some extent. This is a not inconsiderable undertaking when one considers the different and unique background, training, experience, loves, hates, attitudes and personality structure of each partner. Studies have been made which show that, in fact, the choice of a mate is limited. The 'pool' of eligible mates from which one is selected is usually determined by the race, the social class, the age, the level of education, the location of residence, the religion of the candidate. It is true that a few couples step over the expected boundaries and successfully marry outside their 'class' or 'race', but even in multi-racial societies, such as Malaysia and Fiji, inter-racial marriages are unusual.

As well as the 'social factor', there is a second, less-understood factor which has been called the 'complementary need factor'. This factor is much more specific for each individual, and operates usually without their knowing it in their choice of a person with whom 'to fall in love'. A woman who needs to 'mother' another person may choose a man who has an obvious problem, and she gratifies her 'need' for mothering by looking after him and helping him to overcome his problem. An aggressive, demanding man may select a timid, passive woman, on whom he can vent his need for aggression, without receiving a rebuff. These are extreme examples, and the whole matter is not really understood, particularly as many marriages are contracted for emotional rather than rational reasons. In these marriages, it has been suggested that the 'complementary need factor' may operate. The strongly-sexed male may be attracted to a girl who refuses his sexual advances because she is weakly-sexed, or because her upbringing has led her to believe that premarital sex is prohibited. His main reason for seeking marriage may be that she refuses to permit premarital sexual intercourse. Meanwhile he has sexual intercourse with other more highly-sexed girls, but because he subconsciously values virginity, would not think of marrying one of them although she might make him a more suitable partner.

In our society sexual compatibility is an important factor in keeping a marriage stable but, of course, it is only one of many factors. If one of the partners to a marriage has been taught to believe that sexual intercourse is something shameful and dirty, and that for a woman sexual intercourse is something to be passively endured rather than an activity for the mutal pleasure of the couple, problems will arise.

Clearly, incompatibility will not vanish if both husband and wife have received some education in sexual matters, but the problems will be reduced. Obviously, too, a knowledge of sex will not make a wife happier whose husband is an alcoholic or a philanderer. Nor will it keep the marriage stable if the male is brutal, emotionally disturbed or completely selfish. But then any attempt by one individual to bend or damage the personality of another is a sin, if not a legal one, one against humanity, particularly in a marriage where the two personalities are in intimate contact over a long time. Since the sexual side of personality is an important one, perhaps this is the reason why sexual compatibility plays such an important part in a stable marriage. It gives even greater emphasis that 'marriage should be made harder to obtain, and divorce easier'.

The honeymoon

For the minority of the young people who have not experienced premarital sexual intercourse, the honeymoon can be a time of uncertainty. The excitement of the engagement, culminating in an emotionally exhausting wedding and reception, is hardly the most suitable introduction to their first sexual encounter. In our society, the man is more likely to have had sexual intercourse before marriage than the girl. But his experience may well be limited and his technique inadequate. After the wedding, the bride is often anxious, nervous and tired, and the husband clumsy and too forceful in his approach. The main problem is that a woman takes rather longer to arouse sexually than a man, particularly if she is a virgin. The male should spend a rather longer time therefore before he attempts to introduce his penis into her vagina. Kissing, bodily contact like hugging, breast stroking, lightly touching her abdomen and the inner surface of her thighs, and wandering his hand gently to caress her vulva and clitoris, will slowly but surely bring her into a receptive frame of mind. This is shown by increased secretion of the glands just inside the vulva, so that the entrance to her vagina becomes moist. These secretions also act as a lubricant for the penis as it enters the vagina. In passing, it should be noted that if the husband decides to use a condom, he must lubricate it with a jelly ('surgical' jelly is sold in tubes by pharmacists) on the outside, or the first attempt at coitus may be painful.

The psychological dangers of forceful, clumsy attempts at penetration on a wife who is not ready for coitus have been exaggerated. Even so, a traumatic first coital encounter by an insensitive husband may create anxieties in the wife which even her love for him cannot resolve, and their sexual relationship is marred. The full establishment of sexual compatibility may take some time.

Once the girl is aroused, she should gently guide her husband's penis so that it lies against her hymen, making sure that no strands of vulval hair are in between. If she lies on her back, with the husband on top of her, her legs apart, her knees bent, she will find it easier to guide her husband's erect penis. In this position, as he lies over her, he slowly and gently presses his penis into the vaginal entrance, and then withdraws slightly. This movement is repeated, and each time he presses his penis a little further into the vagina, always moving slowly so that the muscles which surround the vagina have time to dilate, and the hymen to stretch. Slowly he moves, and soon he finds that his penis has been introduced fully into his wife's vagina. If he tries to introduce it too quickly, he will cause her pain, and her muscles will contract, causing more pain. But by gentle penetration, coitus can proceed normally, the penis deeply inside the vagina and its thrusting movements bringing the husband to orgasm. Immediately after ejaculation of semen, the tip (or glans) of the penis is exquisitely sensitive, and the erection subsides. The sensitivity lasts only for a few moments, but whilst this is occurring he will lie inert and still, relaxed, upon his wife.

It is possible that she too will reach an orgasm, but this is unlikely, and to relieve her sexual tension he can often bring her to orgasm by lightly stroking her clitoris with his fingers.

Sexual intercourse is repeated as often as the couple desire, and depending on whether or not the wife is sore from previous episodes. Soon, however, the husband will find that the introduction of his penis is much easier, and the muscles around the vagina relax more readily. The couple's sexual relations are beginning to become adjusted. Since it is the girl who has to adjust more, because she is aroused more slowly and is more likely to be a virgin at marriage, the husband must be patient, gentle and considerate in his coital demands. He should let his wife set the pace.

Coitus during menstruation and pregnancy

The belief that sexual intercourse is dangerous during menstruation is erroneous. It is true that it is messy, but the tissues of the vagina are no more fragile at this time, so that there is no reason why the couple should not have sexual intercourse during the wife's menstrual period if they wish, particularly as at this time the wife's desire is often increased. Sexual intercourse can also take place throughout pregnancy if the couple so desire. This is discussed further on p. 159.

COITUS

The introduction of the male sex organ into the body of a female partner is called coitus, or sexual intercourse. The word coitus is derived from the Latin *coitio*, which is made up of *co-*, together, and *ire-*, to go. It means to 'go together'. Although in Christian theology coitus took place mainly for the procreation of children, it was also permitted as an expression of the love that existed between the two marriage partners. Today with contraception, these two functions can be separated, and coitus is increasingly used as a means to relieve sexual tension, to obtain mutual sexual satisfaction, and to show mutual love.

Frequency

Sexual intercourse takes place most frequently in the first years of marriage, often occurring once every 24 hours. The frequency may fall off after one or two years, to two or three times a week up to the age of about 35. As middle age approaches, and the pressures of work increase, at a time when the physical attractions of the spouse are decreasing, coital frequency may fall to once a week or less. There are very considerable variations, and some couples only have sexual intercourse at infrequent intervals in the early years of marriage, whilst other couples copulate frequently and satisfactorily even in old age.

It is sometimes asked, can coitus take place too frequently? The answer is a firm no! There is no such thing as 'excessive coitus', provided the male can obtain and maintain an erection of his penis, and provided that he can do this as often as he and his wife desire to have sexual intercourse, coitus can take place as often as they wish. Frequent coitus does not lead to any weakness of either partner, although it may cause lack of sleep. Occasionally frequent coitus does cause irritation to one or other partner's genitals from over-stimulation or friction. In such cases, a period of a couple of days' rest will restore the function to normal.

What frequency of sexual intercourse is suitable for the couple is normal. 'Excessive' coitus has no harmful effects, and 'infrequent' coitus (if this pattern is acceptable and not frustrating to either partner) is equally innocuous. In fact, frequency of coitus is a matter of personal choice, and what the couple considers normal for them, is normal.

Coital positions

Sexual intercourse can take place in a variety of positions. These have been described in the literature of all cultures, and ancient Indian literature is particularly informative, as shown by Vatsyayana's *Kama-Sutra*, written in 200 B.C., and in the sculptures on the temples of Khajuraho. Basically, the positions can be reduced to about half a dozen, all of which are 'normal'.

Face to face, the man on top: The man lies on top of the woman, either putting his weight upon her, or supporting most of his weight on his elbows or hands. She spreads her legs apart, and may for variety flex her knees, sometimes placing them around her partner's waist. She may place a pillow beneath her buttocks to lift her pelvis. There are many variations of this basic position. The woman may keep her legs stretched out, her partner's legs inside hers, or she may bring her legs together, so that her partner's knees are outside. She may flex her thighs more so that her legs are clasped round his shoulders.

This position is the most usual, and has the advantage that it makes penile entry into the vagina easy; the bodies of the two partners are in close proximity, so that they can kiss and caress each other during coitus; it permits the male to set the pace and slow or hasten coitus, to reach an orgasm at a desired speed; and it is probably the

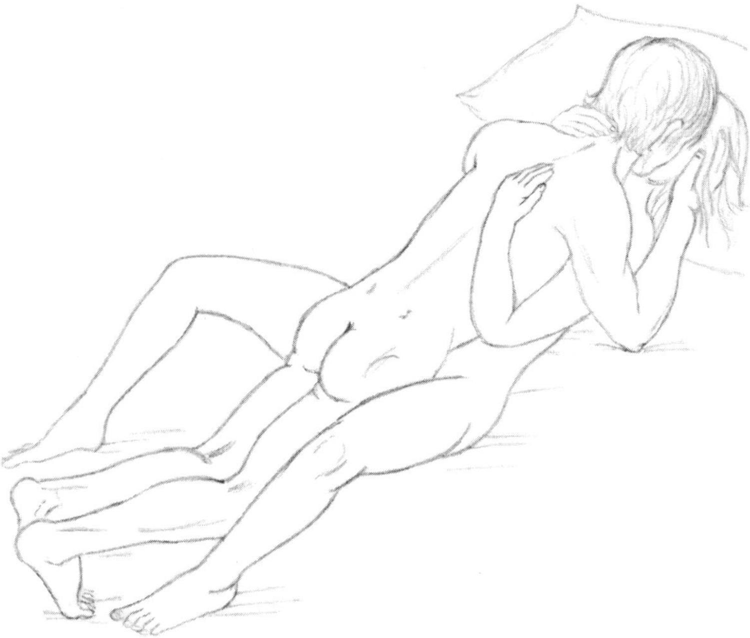

FIG. 5/1. Coital positions. Face to face, man on top

best position for pregnancy to occur, as after ejaculation the seminal fluid bathes the cervix. The disadvantages of the position are that it restricts the woman's movements and thrusts; male orgasm is often reached too quickly; penetration may be painfully deep, and the male is unable to caress the woman's clitoris during coitus, which she may desire.

Face to face, woman on top: The man lies on his back, the woman squats over him and guides his penis into her vagina. Once this has occurred, she may lie upon him, her weight resting on his body; she may support her weight on her arms; or she may sit upright across his thighs. The man may lie flat, raise himself on his arms, or clasp his legs around his wife's waist.

This position is an advantage if the husband is very heavy, his wife light in weight. In it the woman has the greatest freedom of

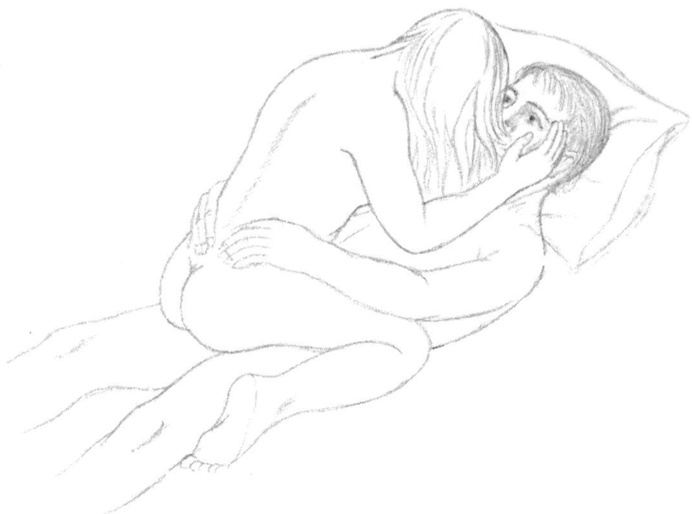

FIG. 5/2. Coital positions. Face to face, woman on top

movement, and the male can caress her clitoris and vulval area during coitus.

The disadvantages are that some women cannot control the depth of penile penetration too easily, and it may be too deep and so painful. During coitus the man's penis may slip out of the vagina, which is uncomfortable for both and spoils smooth coital sequence.

Man's face to woman's back, rear entry: There are several variations of this position. The man may lie behind his wife, his hands around her to caress her breasts or clitoris. She lies in front of him, her legs bent at the hips, her body slightly curved away from his. The man's penis is inserted into his wife's vagina from the rear, and once inside she presses her thighs together and pushes backwards so that her buttocks make a firm contact against his lower abdomen and scrotum. Alternatively, she may lie on her stomach with her pelvis raised and her legs apart. The man lies on top of her, entering her vagina from the rear. Or she may kneel on hands and knees, her

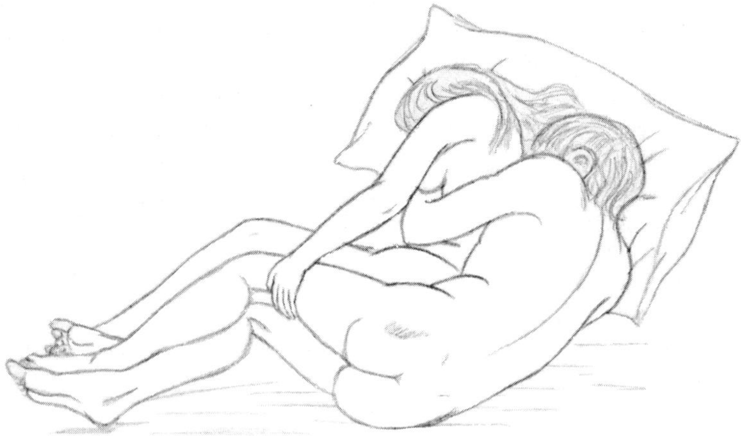

FIG. 5/3. Coital positions. Rear entry

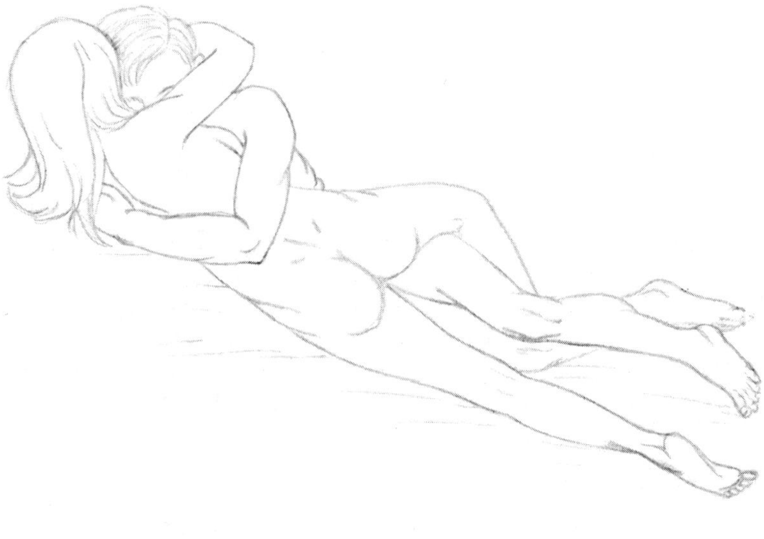

FIG. 5/4. Coital positions. Face to face, side by side

head and breast touching the bed, the man kneeling behind her. In another variation, the man sits on the edge of a chair, or the bed, and his wife, with her back to him, sits upon his penis and as it slips into her vagina, eases herself onto his lap.

The advantages of these positions are that the contact of the woman's buttocks on the man's abdomen, legs and scrotum may stimulate them both; he can readily caress her breasts or her clitoris during coitus; and the couple can rest on their sides during coitus. In late pregnancy, this position is the most suitable one.

Face to face, side by side: This position is, in fact, not exactly side by side, for penile entry would be almost impossible if it were. Usually the couple's legs are interlocked, and the man may lie largely on his back, the woman resting on his chest, or, alternatively, the woman may lie largely on her back, one thigh beneath him.

Sitting positions: The man sits on a chair, or the edge of the bed, and the woman sits astride his lap, his penis within her vagina, his arms around her body, and hers around his. Alternatively, the man can squat behind the woman's thighs, as she lies on her back facing him, with her legs on his hips. He can then make thrusting motions, or pull his wife's pelvis back and forth. Another alternative is for the woman to squat between the man's thighs, supporting her weight on her outstretched arms, whilst he lies on his back with his legs apart. Once his penis is inside her vagina, she moves her pelvis in a circular fashion.

Standing positions: By bending his legs, the man can introduce his penis either facing his wife, or from the rear. She may put her hands around his neck and clasp his hips between her thighs. The couple may move around during coitus, or coitus may take place in surroundings different from normal, such as during a shower.

The advantages of the sitting and standing positions are that they may be more exciting because they are unusual and not used routinely.

Extravaginal coitus

The man may obtain stimulation by rubbing his penis between the woman's thighs, or between her breasts. The sole advantage of these

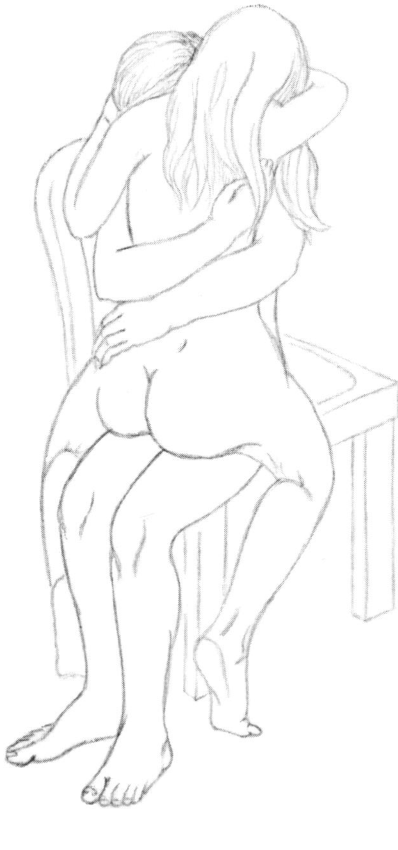

FIG. 5/5. Coital positions. Sitting position

positions, apart from variety, is that the chance of conception occurring is remote, although ejaculation outside the vulva may lead to conception.

One notorious extravaginal position is quite normal and often followed by a deep emotional release. This is the simultaneous caressing of the woman's clitoris and vulva by the man's tongue, whilst she puts his penis in her mouth and caresses it with her tongue until they both have a simultaneous orgasm. Although this position has been condemned by the clergy, and is whispered about by adolescents as the sixty-nine or soixante-neuf position, it is completely normal, and a couple need feel no guilt if they obtain mutual pleasure, happiness, sexual relaxation and release from it.

For sexual intercourse to be truly satisfying, the penile entry into the vagina, or caressing with the tongue, should only come at the end of a sequence of foreplay activities which draw the bonds between the partners closer, surrounding them with feelings of warmth to each other, and joy in their mutual embraces. Sexual intercourse is not just a silent monotonous thrust of an urgent penis into an indifferent vagina. It is a complex, varied group of activities leading to the maximum sexual joy for both participants.

Sexual response in the male

Until recently the response of men and women to sexual intercourse was hidden in a veil of modesty and mystery. A certain sequence of events was known to occur, which led to the ejaculation of semen by the male, and was followed by a warm feeling of release. But what happened in that sequence was unknown until two American scientists, Dr. William H. Masters and Dr. Virginia E. Johnson, investigated the sexual response in both males and females. Since it would be inappropriate to ignore the sexual response of the male, it being so intimately related to that of the female, this is considered first.

The most obvious sign of sexual arousal in the male is the erection of his penis, which enlarges both in length and in its diameter. With further arousal a clear secretion, which may be scanty or profuse, emerges from the 'eye' of the penis and lubricates the glans, whether the man has a foreskin or not. Sexual arousal in the male can be started in several ways, usually by sight or by touch, but each man is stimulated to a different degree. Whilst one man may be sexually aroused by the sight of a girl wearing a tight sweater which emphasizes the size of her breasts, another may be quite indifferent to breast size, but may be markedly attracted to the shape of a girl's legs, her walk or the prominence of her buttocks. Arousal can occur by reading books in which sexual activity is described, or by looking at pictures in magazines. By and large Western man is strongly attracted to and aroused by the breasts and buttocks of the female, whilst in other societies these sexual symbols are not stimulating at all. As well as vision, smell can arouse the male–as every woman knows–which is one of the reasons why she wears perfume, usually sold under a provocatively sexual name. Fantasy, or sexual day-dreaming, can also cause arousal and lead to penile erection, often during sleep.

A much more potent means of sexual arousal is contact with the woman. Kissing, hugging, caressing her breasts are potent arousal stimuli, and may lead to orgasm in themselves, particularly if the woman responds by returning the kisses, by moving her breasts and abdomen against the male, by raising her legs between his, or by stroking his genitals through his clothes. This has been considered in the section on 'Petting'.

Once the penis is in erection, the man is ready for coitus. He has passed through the arousal (or excitement) phase, and has entered what Masters and Johnson call the 'plateau phase'. In erection, the penis approximately doubles its length and measures 9·5 cm. (4 in.). There are several fallacies connected with the penis: the size of the penis is not related to its function. A man with a small penis is as sexually adequate as a man with a large penis, and can provide as much sexual satisfaction to his wife. Another fallacy is that the circumcised male takes longer to reach orgasm, and so may more readily bring his wife to orgasm. The evidence is that there is no difference in time to reach orgasm between circumcised and uncircumcised men. There is, of course, a considerable difference between different men in the time they take to reach an orgasm, but circumcision or its absence is not a factor.

Once penile erection has occurred and the arousal stimulus continues, the man either seeks to have sexual intercourse or masturbates. In essence, there is little difference as far as the penis is concerned. During coitus it is usual for him to thrust his penis in and out of his wife's vagina; during masturbation he stimulates his penis by grasping it lightly and stroking the length of the entire organ.

As orgasm approaches, a time is reached when the man *knows* that within a few moments ejaculation will occur; the phase lasts about three or four seconds, and even if he ceased all movement of his penis, he knows that ejaculation is inevitable. There is nothing he can do to stop it. This time of 'suspended animation' is followed by a warm feeling along the shaft of his penis as the seminal fluid moves from the seminal vesicles, or collecting area, to the tip of the penis. Then spasmodically three to six expulsive contractions of the muscles at the base of his penis lead to spurting of seminal fluid, and simultaneously the muscles of his thighs and lower abdomen jerk and thrust convulsively. During this explosive, expulsive period, he clasps the woman tightly to his body. The 'crisis' passes with smaller contractions fading away. Immediately after ejaculation, the glans of the penis becomes momentarily exquisitely tender, and a feeling of warm well-being surrounds the male. It is usual for complete relaxation and a short sleep to occur (the 'little death' of the French), during which time the penis becomes limp.

Sexual response in woman

As with the male, the sexual response in woman can be arbitrarily divided into four phases, which Masters and Johnson have called (1) the excitement or arousal phase, (2) the plateau phase, (3) the phase of orgasm, and (4) the phase of resolution.

Excitement phase: This phase is initiated more by bodily contact with the male than by visual stimuli, although the sight of an attractive male plays some part. Sexual arousal varies in women depending on the time of the month. Many women have a heightened sexual interest at certain times, often at the midcycle or just before menstruation. But no consistent pattern can be determined. Tradition has held that sexual intercourse during menstruation is dangerous because the tissues are more fragile and liable to infection, but probably really because of the old Jewish law which held a woman to be 'unclean' during menstruation. This is unfortunate because some women are only sexually aroused at this time. There is no medical reason why a woman who desires sexual intercourse during menstruation should not have it. The tissues are *not* more fragile, nor is infection more likely to occur. Coitus is a little messy, but that is all. There is no danger and the woman is *not* unclean.

The excitement phase in the woman tends to be slower to reach its peak, and to last for longer. During it her nipples become erect, and the areola beneath them becomes swollen and dusky. Her clitoris increases in size, mainly in width, and the labia minora become softer and thicker as they become congested with blood. These changes vary in degree from woman to woman. At the same time as these events are occurring, fluid is entering her pelvic tissues, her vagina is becoming softer and some of the fluid seeps through the layers of tiny cells which, like bricks, make up the vaginal wall. The vagina appears to 'sweat' in anticipation of the awaited penis. Two small glands which lie near the opening of the vagina also secrete fluid, so that both the vagina and its entrance become moist and slippery. If the male attempts to introduce his penis before the fluid has been secreted and the area has become moist, coitus will be painful. It is for this reason that the husband should stimulate his wife by kissing her and by stroking her body gently, until she is ready to receive him.

Plateau phase: The woman is now in the 'plateau phase', and is ready and anxious to accept the erect penis into her moist vagina. The thrusting movement of the penis, and the closer physical contact with the male stimulates the clitoral area and the mons veneris, and brings her towards the phase of orgasm. In many instances, though, the man will reach orgasm and will ejaculate before she herself has an orgasm. Frequently she is sexually satisfied by the knowledge that she has been the cause of his pleasure, but sometimes her sexual tension remains high. If this is so, a considerate husband will bring her to orgasm by gently stroking her clitoris and mons veneris.

Orgasm: It has long been believed that woman can have two types of orgasm, the 'clitoral orgasm' and the 'vaginal orgasm'. An error of observation and of deduction by Freud is responsible for this. He maintained that the clitoral orgasm was an immature form, which was obtained by masturbation, and that vaginal orgasm only developed with sexual and psychological maturity, when the centre of sexual sensitivity was transferred from the clitoral area to the vagina. The deduction from this was that masturbation is immature, and the woman who can only reach an orgasm by masturbation is sexually and psychologically immature, whilst the woman who develops a vaginal orgasm is sexually and psychologically mature. This error, although suspected for some time, was finally laid by Masters and Johnson who have shown that an orgasm is an orgasm, and there is no difference in how it is produced, whether as a result of clitoral area manipulation, by movement of the penis in the vagina, or for that matter by simply fondling the breasts.

Orgasm in the female is associated with the same jerking, thrusting movements of the thigh and pelvic muscles, as those of the male. It differs in no way from male orgasm except that there is no ejaculation. During orgasm the muscles of the womb and the vagina contract, and some women have a more intense orgasm if the erect penis is deeply inside the vagina at the time, so that it can be rhythmically gripped and released by the contracting vaginal muscles.

Phase of resolution: As in the male, the convulsive muscle contraction ceases and a feeling of relaxation, relief and sleepiness surrounds and bathes the woman, who may fall asleep. She has entered the phase of resolution. In the initial moments of this phase, the clitoris is exquisitely sensitive (just as is the glans of the penis immediately after ejaculation), but the tenderness rapidly passes and the tissues of the vulva and the vagina lose the fluid which seeped into them over a period of five to ten minutes. The sleep of the resolution phase may last a few minutes or may merge into a sleep lasting hours, depending on the circumstances. If a woman is stimulated to the plateau phase but fails to reach orgasm, the resolution phase is often prolonged and the congestion of the tissues is slow to resolve. Repeated stimulation and failure to achieve an orgasm can lead to physical and mental frustration. It may be the underlying cause of several psychosomatic gynaecological complaints. For this reason as well as for reasons of love and affection, the husband should give his wife an orgasm by caressing her clitoral area, if she desires this. Of course, if she is not stimulated at all, but merely offers herself to her husband so that he may reach an orgasm, she may well be happy that she has made him happy. Since she has not gone beyond the stage of early arousal, she is not distressed by failing to reach an orgasm herself. Over a period of months, she may give her husband many orgasms, but have few herself and be completely content and happy, or she may be frustrated. A few women reach orgasm at every episode of sexual intercourse, and some of these have multiple orgasms during the episodes; but most women only have orgasms occasionally, a few rarely or never.

PAINFUL COITUS (DYSPAREUNIA)

Pain during sexual intercourse is not very common, but can be very disturbing, and indeed if severe can prevent intercourse occurring. The medical term for painful coitus is *dyspareunia.* If a woman has dyspareunia, she should seek medical advice as frequently there is some local condition of the genital organs which causes it. Most of these conditions can be treated easily and quickly, and a woman should not feel ashamed about consulting a doctor. Unfortunately, many women either put up with the pain lest they offend their husbands, or prevent sexual intercourse taking place. It is true that painful intercourse is sometimes psychological in nature, but only after a doctor has made a proper investigation can he say that this is the cause. For example, attempts by the husband to insert his penis into his wife's vagina before she has reached the 'plateau phase', and when the entrance to her vagina is insufficiently lubricated by the normal secretions, can cause marked pain. The normal reaction to pain is to remove oneself from its source, but during coitus this is impossible, so the woman automatically does the next best thing. This is to tighten the muscles around her vagina and its entrance. Of course, this will cause further pain should the husband persist in his attempt, and a habit may develop in which the wife tightens the vaginal muscles when sexual intercourse is attempted. The inability to have normal intercourse makes her believe either that her vagina is too small or her husband's penis is too large, both of these beliefs being false. But even when dyspareunia has a psychological basis, treatment is most satisfactory if the woman seeks it fairly soon after she has found that intercourse continues to be painful or impossible.

REDUCED SEXUAL DESIRE

It was mentioned earlier in this chapter that sexual desire varies very considerably between individuals, but provided the wife and her husband are reasonably similar in their desires, problems do not arise. It was also noted that sexual desire varied during the month, and changed at different times of life. Reduced sexual desire has been called 'frigidity'. This is a bad term for it includes women who have no feeling about coitus, women who are not easily stimulated, women who never have an orgasm, and women who obtain little satisfaction even when they reach orgasm. These women are obviously suffering from different conditions, but in all the underlying problem is a psychological one. A woman is not 'frigid', she has a reduced sexual urge. It is true that certain tranquillizing drugs given to counteract depression are said to reduce sexual interest, but it is very difficult to be sure that the cause of the decline is not the underlying psychological condition rather than the drug.

The exact psychological cause of reduced sexual drive is difficult to distinguish, particularly as most psychiatrists interested in sexual problems tend to disagree amongst themselves, and it takes a great deal of time, energy and enthusiasm to extract the essence of their opinions from the very wordy papers they write.

Three main psychological causes seem to be generally accepted; (1) ignorance of sex, (2) shame about sex, and (3) inadequate relationship with the husband.

IGNORANCE. A considerable number of psychiatrists point out that probably millions of women have a reduced sexual desire due to ignorance. These women believe that they should only submit to their husband's sexual demands, and do not expect themselves to receive any satisfaction. Consequently during coitus their minds are on domestic rather than sexual matters, or are blank. If these women realized that they too should be active partners in sexual activity, and could obtain pleasure, warmth and relaxation from coitus, their sexual desire might well be enhanced.

SHAME ABOUT SEXUAL ACTIVITY. During childhood the girl may be conditioned to believe that sexual activity is something shameful. Sex is never discussed openly, and such information (or more accurately, misinformation) as is obtained, is from whispered confidences from girls of her own age. If the parents consider the human body, apart from the exposed face, arms and legs, to be indecent and punish the girl when she asks about it, or if they do not respond sensibly to the child's natural curiosity about sex and human reproduction, the child is likely to believe that sexual activity is indecent, shameful and something to be ignored as far as possible. This may reflect on her attitudes to sex in marriage.

The opposite attitude towards sex can also occasion shame. The 'sophisticated' girl who has read books about sex and who openly discusses sexual matters may also have a deficient sexual drive. In Western society success is lauded, and if in sexual relations success means consistent orgasm in each episode of sexual intercourse, success may elude many women. This is not because they are inadequate, for as has been stressed, sexual desire (and the ability to achieve an orgasm) varies very considerably during the reproductive years. But because the woman fails to 'achieve success' as shown by orgasm, she becomes ashamed at what she believes is her sexual inadequacy. This shame leads to a reduction in her sexual desire, as a safeguard against 'failure'. During sexual intercourse, a woman can increase her sexual awareness by thinking about sexually arousing stimuli. But if she keeps thinking how terrible it will be, and how inadequate she is if she does not have an orgasm, she may reduce her sexual desire by her over-determination to be a 'normal' woman. This feeling of inadequacy is increased by the cinema and by literature. So many films stress by implication, and so many books indicate explicitly, that when a woman has an orgasm bells ring, lights flash, music falls from the air and the planets stop in their courses, so she believes that she should feel all these things. Yet when an orgasm occurs, a delightful sensation may sweep over her, but there are no fireworks and no comets. She feels, therefore, that she is deficient in femininity, and the conflict engendered by this false belief causes her subconsciously to reduce her sexual desire, to avoid the pain and shame of failure.

If a woman feels shame about sexual activity, she may eliminate this by the knowledge that sexual activity is a normal way of showing love towards a loved one, and that it is unusual for a woman to achieve an orgasm with each coital episode. This in no way means that she is not a normal, healthy woman, with normal attitudes, and the gratification she obtains by *giving* pleasure in itself *gives* her sexual satisfaction. Moreover, if her husband after his orgasm is happy to give his wife an orgasm by manipulation of her clitoral area, her sexual satisfaction is enhanced. In this, too, some women feel shame, believing that an orgasm induced by stimulation of the clitoral area is 'inferior' to an orgasm achieved during penile-vaginal sexual intercourse. Regrettably, many husbands believe that a wife is sexually inferior when she can achieve orgasm only through clitoral caresses. This compounds her shame. These beliefs are wrong scientifically and emotionally. A woman should know that an orgasm is an orgasm no matter how it is produced, that it varies in intensity at different times, and that if no orgasm occurs, she is as sexually adequate as her friends. If she eliminates shame of sex from her mind, her sexual desire will increase.

INADEQUATE RELATIONSHIP WITH THE HUSBAND. In any relationship between two people, and particularly in one as intimate as marriage, conflicts can arise. These conflicts may lead to a change in feeling for the other partner, who is found to be lacking in some expected quality. In this way a woman may become sexually inhibited because she feels her husband no longer cares for her or because she believes she no longer loves him. She may feel that his sexual 'demands' on her are excessive, she may object to certain of his ways of behaviour, or she may resent him (often unconsciously) for things he has or has not done, and the conflict reduces her sexual desire for him.

What can be done?

If the reduction in sexual desire in one or other partner is so great that conflict arises in the marriage, help is needed. This can be given by trained marriage guidance counsellors, who have access to psychiatric opinion should this be required. A couple need feel no shame in seeking help, for it is far better to repair a damaged marriage than to destroy it in silence and antagonism.

In other cases the reduction is far less, and the woman herself can 'train' herself to be roused sexually. If she knows that certain stimuli arouse her sexual desire, she should use these prior to coitus, or involve her husband in what the Americans call 'foreplay to love'. Of course, it means that the husband and wife discuss sexual matters frankly and without any sense of inferiority, guilt or shame. Certain doctors have suggested that if the woman is given male sex hormone injections, her sexual desire increases. There is very little evidence that this is so, and in general these injections should not be given.

NYMPHOMANIA

Whilst increased sexual desire is the normal sexual make-up of some women, an incessant and overwhelming urgency for sexual intercourse, even in the most inappropriate circumstances, is abnormal. This condition is called nymphomania, and it has a psychological basis. Treatment is needed, and should only be given by a qualified psychiatrist who has an especial interest in sexual disturbances.

HOMOSEXUALITY

Over 95 per cent of women find companionship, a stable relationship and sexual fulfilment with a member of the complementary sex. Note that I have called men the complementary sex – not the opposite sex. This is what men are to women, and women to men – the sex of each complements that of the other partner. The remaining 5 per cent of women* have no sexual interest in men (although they may have friends who are men), and their sexual interests, their need for companionship is met by alliance with another woman. These women are homosexuals: their sexual desires are directed to members of their own sex. They are also called lesbians, because a group of homosexual women, prominent amongst whom was the poetess Sappho, lived on the island of Lesbos in the time of the ancient Greek civilization. This civilization, lauded as one of the peak periods of human creativeness, incidentally was relatively permissive in regard to sex.

Until recently it was thought that a homosexual tendency was inborn – in other words, it was there from before birth. Although it is true that there are shades of femininity and masculinity in every person, it is now known that homosexual attitudes are *acquired* during the child's upbringing. It was also thought at one time that feminine men and masculine women were so because the man manufactured too much female sex hormone, and the woman too much male hormone. It is true that women do manufacture some male hormone in a gland called the adrenal, but the quantity is small, and there is no difference in the amount of hormone secreted by

*Kenyon, F. E., Studies of Female Homosexuals, *British Journal of Psychiatry* (1968), **114**, 1337.

homosexual or heterosexual women. A similar consideration applies to men, and the much-derided 'pansy', 'fairy' or 'queer', although different in character, has the same amount of male sex hormone (or androgen) circulating in his blood as the bovine football hero. Very rarely a woman may develop a tumour which manufactures androgen, and as the concentration of androgen increases in her blood, she becomes physically less feminine: hair appears on her body and face, her breasts become smaller, her clitoris enlarges, but her feminine attitudes do not change.

Small children have no particular thoughts about sex–except perhaps to note that little girls do not have a penis–and until parental attitudes direct them into one sexual role or another, they are content, each seeing the other merely as a playmate. However, the cultural attitudes of our society towards sexual differences are soon imposed on the child. Most societies recognize that a distinction between the sexes is needed for survival, and each sex is trained to believe that certain activities are predominantly theirs–housework and cooking are for girls; car-cleaning, wood-cutting, painting are boys' work. In this, societies have capitalized on the Y chromosome, possessed in every male body cell, and absent in every female body cell. There is some evidence that the Y chromosome tends to make men aggressive. It has been found that if a man has two Y chromosomes in each of his body cells (which is a rare defect), he tends to be exceptionally, often criminally, aggressive. But this genetic basis for the way society models its people is only of minor consequence; the upbringing of the child is much more important in forming its sexual attitudes towards the 'normal' sexual attraction to a member of the other sex. Ultimately, then, the sexual inclinations of the child are determined by the attitudes of its parents, and some parents unwittingly encourage homosexuality in their children. These parents would be shocked to learn that this is what they have done, for they are often more rigid in their attitudes, more puritanical towards sex, and more derogatory about homosexuality than average. A brutal father may make his son fearful of men and drawn to his oppressed, humiliated mother, so that he identifies himself with her, and in adult life becomes a passive, 'female type' homosexual. Oddly enough, opposite parental attitudes can encourage homosexuality. The mother who perpetually pampers her son, who never lets him out of her sight, who forbids his playing with 'common, dirty' companions, who surrounds him with 'smother love', may turn him towards homosexuality. This is even more marked when the sex of the child is in some doubt at birth. Since most of these children look like girls, they are brought up as girls, and find that they are quite happy in the female role. Later it may be found that the 'girl' was in fact genetically a male–she had the Y chromosome in all her body cells–but by this time it is almost impossible for her to exchange roles, and unwise for her to be forced to do so unless she wishes it herself.

As far as girls are concerned, it appears that the mother is the dominant parent in the child's sexual development, although a poor relationship with the father is an important factor. The mother who 'wanted a boy but got a girl' may consciously or unconsciously impose her disappointed desire on her daughter, so that in life she has many masculine attitudes. This does not mean that she will become homosexual, but she may. Similarly a mother who has an unhappy relationship with her husband, may influence her daughter to hate men, and later to seek affection and companionship only with women.

The importance of a stable, warm family life as a means of preventing the possible development of homosexuality is shown by a study in Britain of over 120 lesbians. Children reared in families which have only one parent, which are disturbed by distortions in the relationships of the parents to each other or to the child, or whose sexual attitudes are repressive or ignorant, are particularly vulnerable.

In these ways homosexuals are created. Of course, only some children whose backgrounds resemble the ones described become homosexual. Most are normally heterosexual, although their sexuality may be impaired or damaged, so that they find it difficult to achieve a happy relationship with their chosen partner.

Ultimately it is the sensible attitude of the mother to the upbringing of her child which counts. But, as always, the behaviour of both parents towards each other and towards the child influence the way she will develop.

In the normal sexual development of a child, psychiatrists consider that there is a period when homosexual alliances are normal. This period is usually of limited duration during early adolescence, and is marked by a special closeness for a friend of her own sex. For a period, life away from the chosen one is intolerable, the clothes they wear must be the same, they must do the same things, they are miserable when separated. The intense homosexual friendship wanes as the child matures and forms heterosexual companionships. Often it is replaced by a more emotionally stable friendship, which persists throughout life. In some 10 per cent of cases of adolescent homosexual friendship, the sexuality of the girls is stronger than usual, and they mutually masturbate by stimulating each other's clitoris. There need be no parental anxiety about this, as mutual masturbation is without any consequences, and certainly does not predispose to homosexuality in adult life. Another form of the adolescent homosexual phase is the development of a 'crush' or 'pash' for an older person. Again this is a normal phase, and may be less traumatic to the child, and to its parents, than the heterosexual 'crush' on the latest 'pop' or T.V. star which replaces or follows it. Hero-worship is a normal development in which the child, beginning to be independent, sees in the hero a substitute, stronger and more romantic than either a dominating or a cold indifferent parent. The only danger in the homosexual phase of development is that the child may 'freeze' in this phase, and be unable to move on to heterosexual relationships later. This is only likely to occur if its earlier development has been emotionally insecure or disturbed. By the age of 15, the homosexual phase has waned in most girls. They are now more interested in boys; their friendships for other girls lingering on, but with much less intensity. The few who do not develop further remain homosexual.

In our society, female homosexuals are condemned and persecuted far less than male homosexuals. There are several reasons for this. Homosexuality in the male is thought more of a danger to a male-dominated society, where 'men are strong and dominant' and women 'weak and submissive', than is lesbianism. In our culture, women are permitted to show greater physical intimacy between each other than men: girls habitually hug and kiss; if men do this, it is considered improper. For these reasons, female homosexuals may live together in complete intimacy without incurring the disapproval of the community. Male homosexuals living together are sometimes sneered at and attacked. It is true that male homosexuals appear to be less able to form stable associations with each other, and tend to change partners or seek new sexual contacts more frequently than female homosexuals, who are generally 'monogamous' with one partner. This gives some point to society's condemnation of male homosexuals, even if most of it is due to ignorance, prejudice and perhaps to unsolved sexual problems amongst those who condemn. Those who protest too much, may themselves be latent homosexuals, or so psychiatrists believe.

Many female homosexuals can form a stable, happy relationship with another woman, and can lead full, contented lives. These women need no help, and are not a cause for anxiety. Not all are as lucky as this, and some 25 per cent of lesbians have considerable emotional problems. These arise partly because of their own impaired personality development, but more because society's condemnation increases their insecurity, and they need compassion and tolerance rather than derision and disapproval. Homosexuality is due to a defect in personality development. Many heterosexuals have personality problems which cause distress in their sexual relationships, but they are not singled out for disapproval on legal, social, moral or religious grounds. It seems unjust that homosexuals should be, when understanding and sympathy for the girl as a person, not as a lesbian, is what is needed. In the adolescent whose homosexual phase persists with increasing emotional conflicts, psychiatry can help, but the extent to which it will help differs with each individual. However, if the emotional problem is real, it is worth a try.

CHAPTER 6

The infertile marriage

It is a strange thing that in a world where one of the main problems facing mankind is the 'population explosion', or the birth each year of too many children, a fairly large group of women are seeking desperately to become pregnant. In times past barrenness was always blamed on the wife, but today it is known that in many cases the reason for the childlessness lies with the husband.

If a couple are normally fertile, and have sexual intercourse reasonably regularly, a pregnancy will result within one year of marriage in 90 per cent of cases. For this reason, a couple is considered to be infertile after this time, and will require investigations, tests and treatment if they wish to have a child. With treatment about 35 per cent of the infertile couples will achieve their desire–a pregnancy. In recent years the numbers of tests, investigations and suggested treatments have increased very considerably, but the success rate after the investigations has remained stubbornly at the same 35 per cent.

This is not to say that an infertile couple should not be investigated. It is well worth while, but neither the enthusiasm of the doctors, nor the couple's desire to clutch at every straw should lead them on the round of visits to many doctors in many places to receive a variety of treatments to achieve nothing.

Careful investigation of the causes of infertility have shown that in about 25 per cent of cases the wife is at fault, in about 25 per cent of cases the husband. In the remaining 50 per cent of cases factors which affect them both are present.

It is usual for the wife to consult the doctor first when pregnancy fails to occur. This is correct and proper, for it is she who will carry the growing baby in her uterus for the 40 weeks of pregnancy. At this first visit the doctor enquires about the past operations and illnesses she may have had, about her present health, and about her menstrual history. He will want to know when menstruation first started, of its duration, the interval between periods, and if the periods were painful. Also he will enquire about the couple's sexual habits. The patient should not be embarrassed at this, for it is essential for the doctor to know the frequency of sexual intercourse, and whether the wife felt it to be satisfactory. It is then usual for him to examine the woman thoroughly, firstly to make sure she has no disorder which would make pregnancy hazardous to her, and secondly so that he may perform a pelvic examination to make sure that her genital organs are normal, as far as he can tell from this examination. In several surveys of infertile couples, it was found that in 3 per cent sexual intercourse had not taken place properly, and the wife was still a virgin. It was hardly surprising that pregnancy had not resulted!

The doctor will now outline what he intends to do. He will explain that investigation of infertility usually takes about five visits, and that as the problem concerns the husband as much as the wife, he would like to see him as well as her at the next visit.

INFERTILITY FACTORS

The factors which may lead to infertility are rather complex, but can be understood if a little thought is applied. The male seeds, or spermatozoa, have to be ejaculated into the upper vagina. They then wriggle their way through the cervix, swimming up between the seaweed-like strands of mucus which stretch downwards from the cells which line the cervical canal. They have to negotiate the cavity of the uterus, and by the time they have done this, of the millions ejaculated, only hundreds remain active. They then have to get through the narrow opening joining the cavity of the uterus and the hollow tube of the oviduct. Only a few dozen spermatozoa succeed in doing this. They then swim along the oviduct, against the current as it were, to reach the outer portion. If this occurs just at the time when the ovum has been expelled from the ovary, and if the ovum has been taken up by the fine finger-like projections at the end of the oviduct, conception may occur. If it does, the fertilized egg has to pass down the oviduct again, spending three days in the process, during which time it has divided and the one original cell is now a collection of cells, still within the shell of the *zona pellucida*. The fertilized egg reaches the cavity of the uterus three days or so after conception, and then by shedding the zona pellucida, implants itself into the soft, juicy lining of the uterine cavity. If all goes well, it now grows and becomes a baby; if all does not go well, an abortion occurs, which may or may not be noticed by the woman. It has been calculated that where no bar to conception is present and where every chance of becoming pregnant has been taken, in any one month of 100 fertile women, 60 will become pregnant and 40 will not. Of the 60 who do become pregnant, 45 deliver a live baby and 15 abort, but in 6 the abortion is undetected as it happens so early.

Considering the long journey made by the sperm to fertilize the egg, and the long journey made by the fertilized egg to reach the uterine cavity and implant itself there, it is surprising how readily pregnancy occurs. This description of how fertilization takes place enables a list of factors which prevent fertility to be made.

The male factor

The husband may fail to manufacture any spermatozoa, or because of illness which has damaged the tube (the *vas deferens*) linking his testicles to the collecting areas (or *seminal vesicles*) in his prostate gland, the spermatozoa may fail to reach the collecting areas (Fig. **6/1**). The spermatozoa may be few in number or weak in activity, so that they have not the strength to swim up the genital tract of the wife. Finally, the husband may not be able to ejaculate, or even to practise sexual intercourse properly. Because of these possibilities, the doctor enquires from him about any illness he may have had, particularly mumps which may have damaged the testicles, and gonorrhoea which may have damaged the vas deferens. He will also ask about his smoking and drinking habits, for excessive smoking and too much alcohol both reduce sperm production and reduce the frequency of coitus. He will require to know his occupation, for some jobs reduce sperm production; and about his sexual habits. He will perhaps require to examine the husband, although this can be avoided if the husband is embarrassed provided that the doctor is supplied with a specimen of the husband's semen. Three methods are usual for this. The husband may masturbate in the laboratory (a quiet secluded room is provided!) and give the specimen directly to the technician, or he may have coitus with his wife early in the morning. Just prior

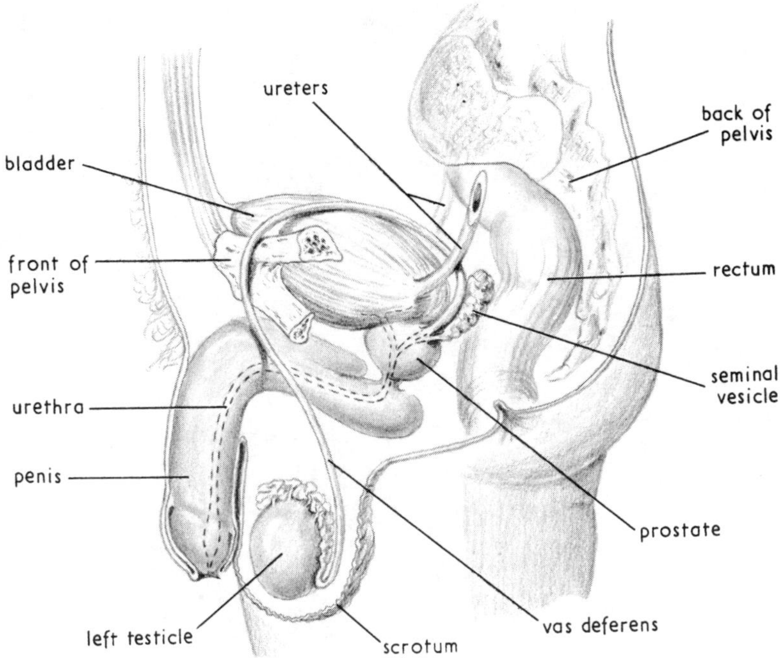

FIG. 6/1. The male genital tract

to ejaculation, he withdraws his penis from his wife's vagina, and ejaculates into a dry, wide-mouthed jar placed beside the bed. His specimen is then brought to the laboratory by the wife, if this is more convenient. The wife should note the time the specimen was produced and bring it to the laboratory within two hours. The final method is not quite so satisfactory, but is preferred by some patients and some doctors. In the third method, the husband and wife have sexual intercourse normally. Six hours later the wife goes to the doctor, who introduces a speculum into her vagina and takes a sample of the semen which is in her vagina (Fig. **6/2**). This method, called the 'post-coital' test, has one particular advantage, it *proves* that normal coitus takes place, although it is much more difficult to determine the quality of the semen from it. And that is the purpose of the test–it is to decide about the quality of the male semen. If it is of poor

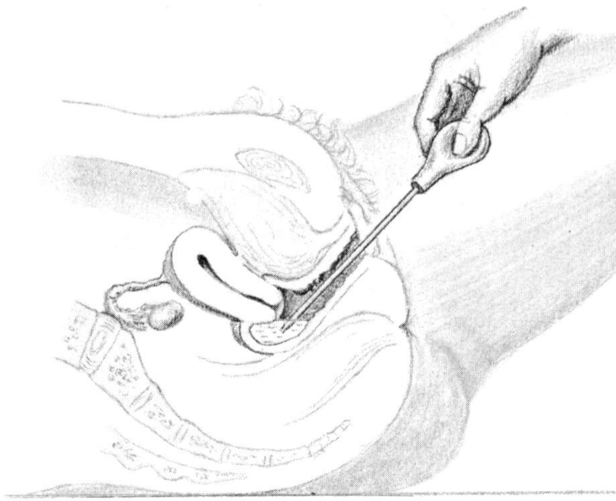

FIG. 6/2. The post-coital test

quality, the test is repeated at least twice, sometimes after giving antibiotics, before any final decision about its quality can be made. Unfortunately, if there are no spermatozoa on all of the tests, the husband is sterile and nothing can be done. If, however, there are spermatozoa but they are of poor quality, certain treatments are available. The man may have varicose veins around his vas deferens, for example. It has been found that the surgical treatment of these varicose veins is often effective in producing a better quality semen. If the husband has no varicose veins, changes in living habits, in tobacco and alcoholic consumption may help. Unfortunately, none of the many hormones, drugs and vitamins which have been prescribed in the past to improve a man's fertility have any effect, whether given by injection or by mouth.

Because it is so easy to check the male factor by examining the semen, this is usually one of the first tests made when infertility is investigated. Indeed, logically a semen analysis should be made before any complicated tests are made on the wife. For example, if the husband were found to be sterile, it would be pointless to perform tests on the wife.

The ovulation factor

Quite obviously if the wife fails to produce an egg, pregnancy cannot occur. Although in the years before the age of 18 and after 38 ovulation occurs less regularly, between these years most women ovulate each month. This can be checked by the wife herself, after consultation with her doctor. Usually she is asked to take her temperature each morning on waking, before she gets out of bed or drinks anything. In a menstrual cycle during which ovulation occurs, the temperature rises in the second half of the cycle. If the daily temperature is charted, this rise can be seen, and the fact of ovulation can be established (Fig. **6/3**). The doctor may use other methods to

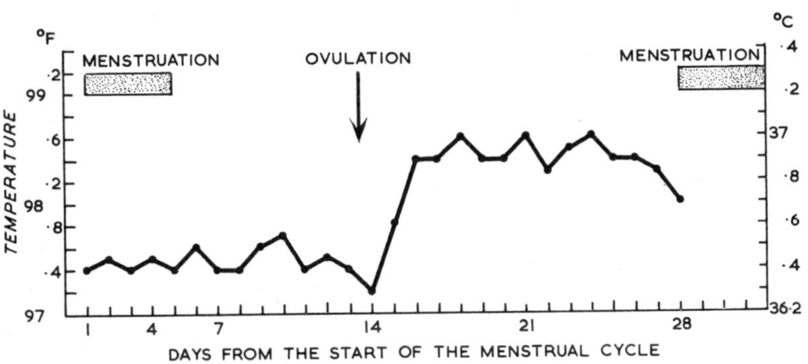

FIG. 6/3. A temperature chart showing that ovulation has occurred on day 14

determine ovulation, and if lack of ovulation is confirmed over several months, one of the special new 'ovulating drugs' may be prescribed, provided no other reason for the couple's infertility has been found. The use of the 'ovulating drugs' is fairly complicated, and most doctors insist that they are only given by specialist gynaecologists who have access to special laboratories, so that the exact dose required for the particular patient may be determined.

The oviductal factor

The sperm has to pass upwards along the oviduct to reach the egg, and the fertilized egg has to pass downwards along the oviduct to reach the uterine cavity. If the oviduct is blocked, these essential events cannot happen. The next step in the investigation, after the husband has been found to be normal, and the wife to be ovulating, is to determine if the oviducts are clear. This is done by blowing a gas through the oviducts. A small tube is placed in the cervical canal, and with a piece of equipment carbon dioxide gas is blown through the uterus and the oviducts. If the gas fails to pass through, this fact can be recorded (Fig. **6/4**). Failure of gas to pass may merely mean that the oviducts are in spasm, and further tests are carried out. The

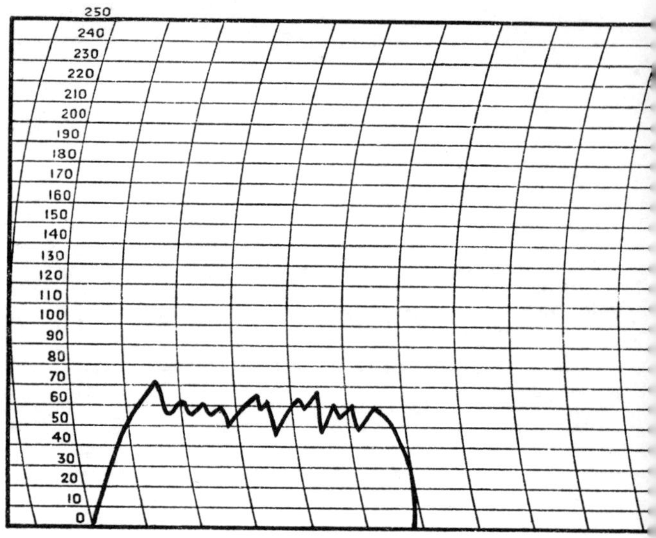

FIG. 6/4. Tracings of a 'gas test' on the oviducts: pressure in mm. of mercury
(a) The gas passed through the oviducts after a pressure of 70 mm. mercury

gas-test may be done without any anaesthetic, when it is slightly uncomfortable, or under anaesthesia. If a block in the oviduct is suspected, a further gas-test is done a month or so later, or an oily substance is injected through the cervical canal and X-rays are taken. These outline the shape of the uterine cavity, and show if either, or both, of the oviducts is 'blocked', and where it is blocked.

Other tests

In certain cases other complicated tests are done, and surgical operations may be required. One of the most difficult problems is when the only reason for infertility is found to be blockage of the oviducts. Surgery may help here, but is best performed by a gynaecologist who makes a special study of infertility surgery. Even in his hands, only one woman in seven who is operated upon succeeds in having a live baby, although one in four succeeds in getting pregnant.

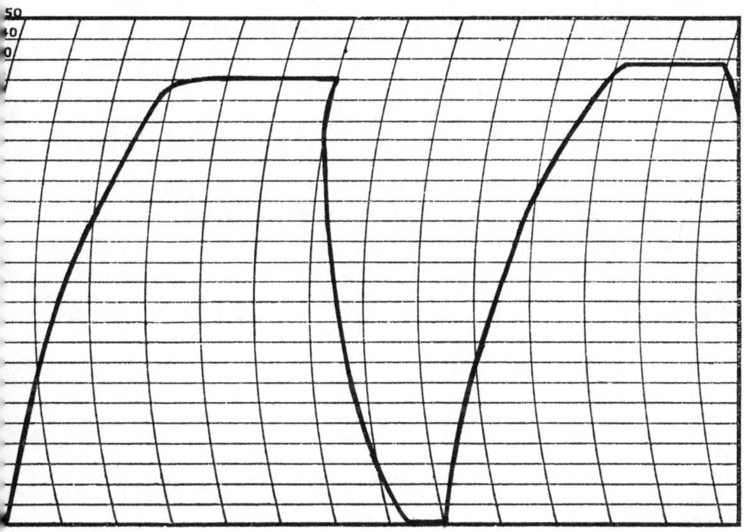

(b) The gas failed to pass through the oviduct despite a pressure of 220 mm. mercury

ARTIFICIAL INSEMINATION OF DONOR'S SEMEN

It may be that the only reason for the barrenness of the couple is that the husband is sterile. In these circumstances, some couples decide that they would prefer to let the wife bear the child of an unknown donor's semen, rather than adopting a child or doing nothing at all. The characteristics of the husband are matched as closely as possible to the unknown donor. He is never seen, or known, by the couple, nor does he know to whom his donated semen has been given. At about ovulation time, the wife goes to the doctor's surgery and each day for three or four days the donor's semen is injected into her upper vagina to bathe the cervix. This is called artificial insemination of donor's semen, or A.I.D. On an average about four inseminations are needed to obtain a pregnancy, and about half the women inseminated become pregnant and deliver a live child. This child is brought up as the natural child of the father. The legal position of the child is not quite clear, and a couple who decide after careful thought to try A.I.D. should take legal advice.

Infertility investigations take time and pose problems. Because of this, the couple must co-operate fully and should seek a doctor who has an interest in infertility, who is sympathetic to the patients, and who is careful never to do too much to little purpose. Although 35 per cent of couples will achieve a pregnancy, it is kinder to tell some of the others that pregnancy is impossible, and to suggest adoption whilst they are still relatively young. An adopted child can give as much joy to a family as a natural child.

CHAPTER 7

Family planning

A fertile woman, having every opportunity to conceive, has a 60 per cent chance of becoming pregnant in any one month if she takes no steps to prevent conception. Each day, all over the world, many women become pregnant, and because medical science has been able to reduce the deaths of infants and children, the population is increasing rapidly. In the year 1770, the population of the world was an estimated 1,000 million; in 1880 it had risen to 1,500 million; by 1980 it will be 4,000 million. To put this another way, it took from man's emergence on this earth until 1805 for the world's population to reach 1,000 million; it took just over 150 years–to 1955–for it to double to 2,000 million; yet in only 25 years–that is by 1980–it will have doubled again to 4,000 million (Fig. **7/1**).

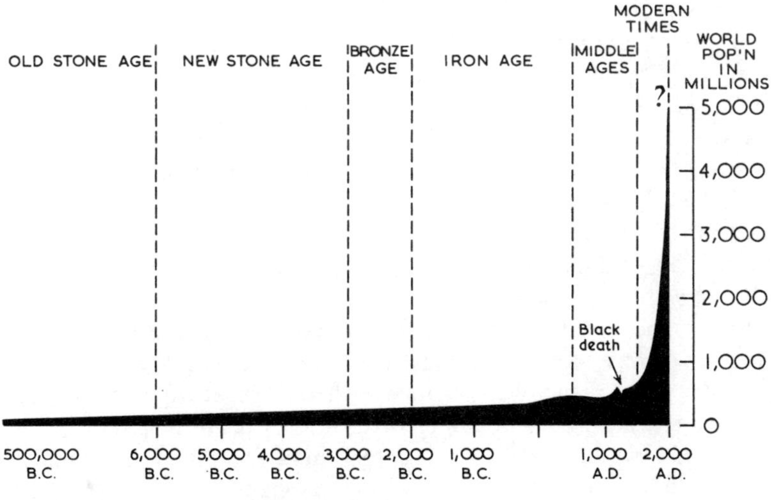

FIG. 7/1. The growth of the world's population, redrawn from *Population Bulletin*, **18**, 1, 1962

This is what the experts call the 'population explosion', and unfortunately the greatest increases, and the highest birth rates, are occurring to the women of the developing countries of the world. In these lands, there is even today too little food for everybody to have sufficient to eat, there are not enough jobs for everyone to have work, and far too much misery and poverty affects the majority of the population.

Unless the world as a whole can increase food production and its equitable distribution, can stimulate trade, can suppress national jealousies, and can stop the 'population explosion' as quickly and efficiently as possible, a disaster foretold over 150 years ago by that gloomy economist, Dr. Malthus, may overwhelm us all. In the words of a Director-General of the United Nations Food and Agricultural Organization, 'Mankind will be overtaken by the old Malthusian correctives–famine, pestilence and war'.

The problem in the developing countries is a national one to curb their population growth or face disaster. The problem for the individual woman, whether in the developing or affluent countries, is a personal one. A new pregnancy may be greeted with joy, as a long-awaited, much-wanted event, or it may appear a disaster to be coped with and overcome. In most Western societies it is a disaster if the mother is unmarried. Unmarried mothers are considered to have loose morals, to be unstable, undeserving and undesirable (whilst the unmarried father gets away with it!). There are exceptions, such as the Scandinavian countries, where unmarried mothers are treated by society in a much more rational and kind way. But in most of the West, pregnancy in an unmarried girl is considered a disgrace.

Even if the woman is married, the new pregnancy may mean that her other children will have less food, a smaller opportunity for education. or that the house will be more crowded. Whatever the reason. she may not want the baby. Both the unmarried mother and the married woman may seek to have the pregnancy ended–to have an abortion induced. whether legally as in some countries. or illegally as in most others. Illegal abortion is also known as 'criminal abortion'. or induced abortion. It is a poor, ineffectual way to deal with the problem of unwanted pregnancies. It would be far, far better for the pregnancy to be *prevented*, not terminated. Yet induced abortion is probably the most usual way of population control in the world today, especially in South America, Eastern Europe and parts of East Asia.

Because women must seek the induced abortion, whilst the man who made her pregnant escapes involvement, induced abortion is discussed here. Of all social problems, those of abortion and of conception control are the most urgent to solve in this decade. They cannot be solved by men alone; they can only be solved by men and women thinking and working together.

THE PROBLEMS OF INDUCED ABORTION

Induced abortion to control the size of a woman's family has been employed for as long as recorded history. In the days when children were necessary to safeguard the family's survival, when they added to its prestige, and were needed to support the parents in their old age, it is likely that only unmarried women sought abortions. This situation no longer applies in modern society, since medicine has reduced the death rate dramatically, and so in recent years both married and unmarried women have visited abortionists to have unwanted pregnancies terminated. In Britain, for example, before the recent Abortion Act which made legal abortions more freely available, it was calculated that over 80,000 illegal abortions took place each year, and that in the majority of cases it was the unmarried girl who sought illegal abortion. Although fewer than 5 of every 10,000 women died following the abortion, many women bled excessively, some became infected, and many suffered serious guilt as a result of the operation.

These considerations were responsible for the introduction in 1968 of a new Abortion Act, under which a woman might have her pregnancy terminated in hospital (or in a few registered nursing homes) for specific medical reasons, which are described in the Act, or for the reason 'that the continuance of the pregnancy would involve risk of injury to the physical or mental health of any existing children of the pregnant woman's family greater than if the pregnancy were terminated'. Since the Act was passed, about 600 legal abortions have taken place each week in Britain. Although it appears that fewer illegal, or criminal, abortions are being performed, the number must be considerable as in the first year since the Act 35 women died following suspected criminal abortions. In the same year, 6 women died after legal abortions.

Japan, facing a rising population with limited land and jobs, introduced legalized abortion in 1949. It is estimated that one-third of all Japanese women have had at least one abortion, and the birth rate has dropped very considerably. In the last 10 years about one million abortions have been performed each year.

In the Eastern European countries, legal abortion is allowed 'on demand', and in Hungary between 1960 and 1964 more legal abortions were performed than babies born. Of every 100 pregnancies, 10 aborted spontaneously, 50 were aborted legally, and 40 ended with the mother delivering a live-born baby.

In countries where legal abortion is condemned, such as the South American countries, it has been calculated that one-third of all hospital beds are occupied by women who have had illegal abortions performed, mostly by 'backstreet' abortionists. Illegal abortions account for nearly half of all deaths of pregnant women, and many of the surviving women become sterile because infection introduced during the procedure has damaged their oviducts.

HOW AN ABORTION IS PROCURED

Many ways have been suggested, and tried, by women to procure an abortion on themselves. Women have tried lying in very hot baths, drinking gin, jumping off tables for hours on end, taking hormone tablets, taking strong purgatives, and taking large doses of quinine. All fail. The only successes were when the woman thought she might have been pregnant, and the worry had delayed her menstrual period. This convinced her that she was pregnant, so she used one of the methods mentioned. This appeared to work, but in fact she was never pregnant in the first place. If a woman is pregnant, none of the methods work.

However, if a girl has been silly enough to try any of the medicines mentioned, and although they have made her feel very ill (which they do) and have not provoked an abortion, she can be assured that they will not have harmed the fetus. If she decides that she will go on with the pregnancy, the baby will not have been damaged in any way.

Because of the ineffectiveness of the 'home remedies', most women who want pregnancies terminated go to abortionists. The 'backstreet abortionists' usually introduce some object through the cervix into the womb. The cheapest ones use wooden sticks; the more proficient ones, who usually have some slight knowledge of medicine, use instruments. Both are dangerous, as the visit is hurried, cleanliness inadequate, and the risks of the mother bleeding severely or becoming infected are great. Higher up the scale are the 'professional abortionists'. Their fees are higher, and they may be qualified doctors. Because of greater knowledge of hygiene and of the techniques involved in procuring an abortion, they are generally much safer. The abortion is obtained by introducing an instrument through the cervix into the cavity of the uterus, and either gently scraping the conception sac from its attachment to the wall of the womb, or by sucking it out with a special suction apparatus, which is like a miniature vacuum-cleaner. The relatively few women dying or developing serious infection following termination of pregnancy by a 'professional abortionist' suggests that in their hands the operation is fairly safe, if expensive. Even in countries where abortion is illegal, pregnancy may be terminated by qualified doctors for certain conditions, if not legally, at least with the Law closing its eyes. The nature of the conditions varies, but in most countries psychiatric reasons head the list, with other medical diseases far behind. This form of induced abortion is called a 'therapeutic abortion', and it is done to save the mother's life or to preserve her health. It is said, somewhat unfairly, that if you want an abortion and have the money, you obtain a psychiatrist's opinion and the abortion is 'therapeutic'; but if you are poor, you go to the 'backstreet abortionist'. In countries which have a more liberal attitude to abortion, abortion may be 'legally' performed on demand (as in Hungary), or if the patient can meet certain conditions (as in Britain).

In many countries there is a demand that the laws regarding abortion should be made more liberal. This has a danger. Unless the campaign to liberalize the abortion laws is preceded by a campaign to give every woman the knowledge of the advantages of contraception, and the facilities to obtain contraceptives easily, more liberal abortion laws may lead to abuse. It is surely far better to prevent pregnancy by contraception, than to sacrifice an unwanted fetus by aborting it. Provided women have the facilities to obtain contraceptives, and are motivated to use them, liberalized abortion laws can be beneficial for those women who become pregnant inadvertently, and who do not wish to continue the pregnancy.

CONCEPTION CONTROL

Pregnancy can be prevented by prohibiting the spermatozoon from reaching the egg, by preventing the egg from being released from the ovary, by hurrying the passage of the egg along the oviducts, or by so altering the lining of the womb that it will not permit the fertilized egg to implant itself. One or more of these methods are used for control of conception, or family planning as it is usually called.

Since population control is now of such importance, and is made a matter of policy by many Governments, it has been found useful to compare the efficiency of the various methods of preventing pregnancy. The measure of efficiency which is used by many people is called the Pregnancy Index, or Rate. This is calculated in the following way:

$$\frac{\text{The number of pregnancies} \times 1{,}200}{\text{Total months of exposure to pregnancy}}$$

The result is expressed as the number of pregnancies 'per hundred woman years', or per 1,200 months of exposure. This rate shows how often in every 1,200 months a woman may expect to become pregnant, or how many of every 100 women using the particular method will become pregnant if they use the method for one year.

Contraceptive measures can therefore be used by the man or by the woman, but usually today the woman takes the measures. However, every educated woman should know of all available methods, and so measures which may be used by the man will also be considered.

Contraceptive methods used by the man

THE CONDOM: If the male covers his penis with a sheath, which is so thin that it is not noticed by husband or wife, but so strong that neither the movement of the penis in the vagina, nor the ejaculation of semen tears it, pregnancy will be prevented as no spermatozoa will be deposited near the cervix. The sheath (or condom), which is today made of fine latex rubber, has been used since Roman times (Fig. **7/2**). In the past century its use has been widespread, and although primarily used to prevent conception, the condom was

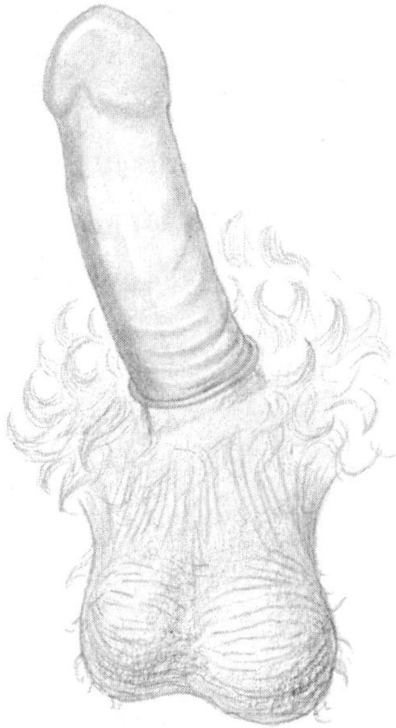

FIG. 7/2. The condom drawn onto the erect penis

issued to soldiers who were going to fornicate with prostitutes as a method of preventing them from catching venereal disease. If the penis was 'protected' by the condom, the germs which live in the genital tract of many prostitutes were unable to get into the delicate tissues of the opening of the 'eye' of the glans of the penis, or to invade the glans itself. In this way the spread of gonorrhoea and syphilis was to some extent prevented.

The disadvantages of the condom, or French letter, as a method of contraception are that the male must put it on, usually waiting until he has an erection of his penis. The need to do this may interfere with his love-making, and he may therefore decide 'to take a chance'. The condom is also expensive, as it is thrown away after being used once. However, it has a considerable popularity, particularly in India where cheap Government-sponsored condoms are issued to men in an effort to reduce the number of babies born. The pregnancy rate amongst the wives of users of condoms is 15 per 100 woman years.

TYING THE VAS: A more permanent method of population control, which can only be used by men who have decided that their family is as large as they want, is to tie the vas deferens, the tube which carries the spermatoza from the testis to the collecting area (Fig. **7/3**).

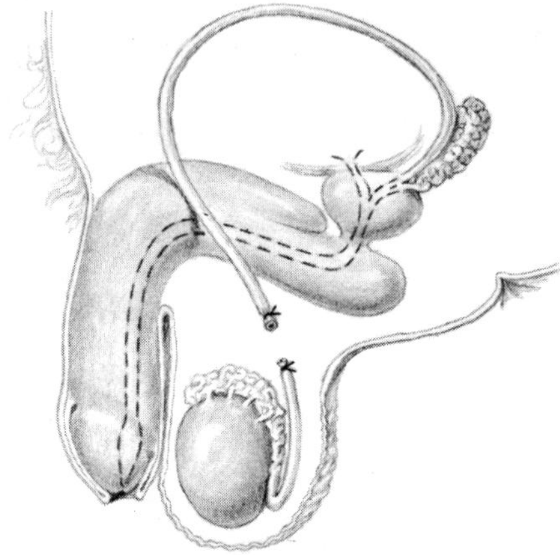

FIG. 7/3. Ligation of the vas deferens

After the operation spermatozoa continue to be made, but the man is sterile. The operation is done under a local anaesthetic through tiny incisions on each side of the upper part of the scrotum, or bag, in which the testicles lie. After the operation, the man finds his sexual desires are unaltered, but no further children are born to his wife, at least after the spermatozoa which were in his seminal vesicles have been ejaculated. This is thought to occur after about six orgasms.

In India a campaign has been conducted since 1964 to induce men to have a 'vasectomy'–or tying of the vas–performed. About 10 million men have been operated upon. The men are given money to compensate for the 4 days they must take off work, with a little over.

COITUS INTERRUPTUS: For many years withdrawal of the penis from the vagina just before ejaculation has been used to avoid pregnancy. In several investigations, made in the days before the Pill became available, it was found to be the most usual method adopted. It relies, of course, on the ability of the man to recognize the sensations which occur in his genitals just before ejaculation, and for him rapidly to withdraw his penis from the vagina and ejaculate outside. This requires great self-control, as the man will often want to keep his penis in his wife's vagina for as long as possible to obtain the greatest amount of pleasure. As the first spurt of semen, which contains the most spermatozoa, may either be ejaculated during withdrawal or may spurt into the vaginal entrance, the risk of pregnancy is high, and the pregnancy index is 35 per 100 woman years.

Coitus interruptus has been said to lead to pelvic discomfort in the wife, who is stimulated but not relieved, and in the husband who has to withdraw at a moment when he would penetrate more deeply. Over long periods it was said to cause mental disorders. There is no evidence that coitus interruptus leads to either of these diseases, or indeed to any disease at all, but it is not a very satisfying method for either husband or wife. Better methods are available.

Contraceptive methods needing the co-operation of both partners

The only contraceptive method at present accepted by the Roman Catholic Church is the *rhythm method*. The method relies on three facts, which may or may not be completely accurate in humans. Firstly, ovulation only occurs once in a menstrual cycle, and if the egg is not fertilized, it will only survive for about 72 hours. Secondly, the single ovulation takes place 13 to 15 days before the first day of the next menstrual period. Thirdly, the spermatozoa can only survive for about 72 hours in the genital tract of a woman. If the couple abstain from coitus at the time of supposed ovulation, and for 3 days on each side, pregnancy should not occur. The rhythm method demands the co-operation of both partners, and coitus is dictated by the calendar rather than by desire. Unfortunately, the rhythm method is not very successful in preventing pregnancy, as ovulation may occur at other times in the cycle, especially if the emotions are stirred. The second reason why the rhythm method fails is that a woman can only establish the approximate time when she will ovulate by recording six menstrual cycles, calculating the day of ovulation in the shortest and longest cycles, subtracting 3 days from the ovulation day in the shortest cycle and adding 3 days to the ovulation day in the longest cycle. The couple should abstain from coitus subsequently in any menstrual cycle on the days which have a 'risk of pregnancy' (Fig. **7/4**). The calculation is fairly complex, as can be seen, and the safe days are few. Attempts have been made to predict ovulation by having the woman take her temperature

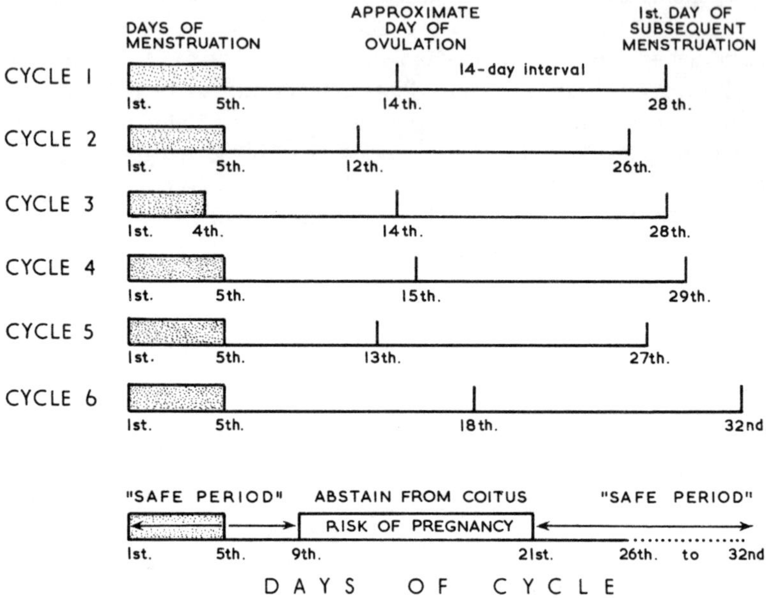

FIG. 7/4. The Rhythm Method: calculation of the 'Safe Period'. In this example the shortest cycle was 26 days, the longest was 32 days. Ovulation in the shortest cycle was calculated to take place on day 12, in the longest on day 18. Three days each side of ovulation are potentially fertile (as the spermatozoa and ovum live for 3 days). For this particular woman, the days on which coitus should be avoided are from day 9 (i.e. the day of ovulation in the shortest cycle, less 3 days) to day 21 (i.e. the day of ovulation in the longest cycle, plus 3 days).

each morning, and noting the rise of temperature indicating impending ovulation. Unfortunately the method is not reliable, and anyhow if coitus has taken place on the day before the rise, the spermatozoa may still be active when ovulation occurs on the following or subsequent day.

Although the safe days are not numerous, coitus can take place quite safely during menstruation, in fact many women experience an increase in sexual desire during this time. The pregnancy rate using the rhythm method is about 30 per 100 woman years.

Contraceptive methods used by the woman

DOUCHING: Many women believe that if they douche immediately after coitus, they will prevent pregnancy occuring. There is no truth in this belief, as the spermatozoa enter the cervix almost immediately after ejaculation. The douche only washes the vagina, and clears the semen left there. Moreover, nothing can spoil sexual relationships more than the wife leaving the bed immediately after her husband's orgasm to go and douche. Douching is a poor method of contraception on all counts.

VAGINAL JELLIES OR CREAMS: These are preparations containing chemicals which will kill spermatozoa if the sperms are in contact with the chemical for sufficient time. Used alone, the jelly (which may foam) is introduced high into the vagina with a tube and plunger, just prior to coitus. It is a poor method of contraception. Spermicidal jellies are also used in conjunction with vaginal diaphragms, and in this they have great value.

THE VAGINAL DIAPHRAGM: As its name implies, the vaginal diaphragm, or Dutch cap, consists of a thin rubber dome which has a coiled metal spring in the rim. The diaphragms are made in various sizes, and the patient must be fitted with the size most suitable for her vagina. She is taught to smear spermicidal jelly in the dome and around the rim of the cap, and to insert it into her vagina by squeezing it. Usually she squats, or stands with one foot on a chair, to introduce the cap, and inserts it into her vagina in an upward and backward direction. Inside the vagina, it regains its shape and fits snugly across the vagina covering the cervix (Fig. **7/5**).

The woman should insert the diaphragm every night routinely, whether or not she expects to have sexual intercourse. The diaphragm is left in place for about 6 hours after coitus, and then removed and washed. If coitus does not take place or occurs before going to sleep, it is removed in the morning; but if the couple copulate in the morning, the diaphragm is left in the vagina until evening.

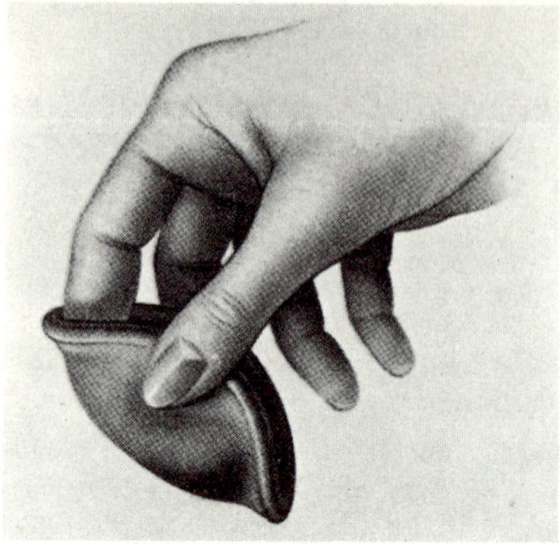

(a) Holding the diaphragm

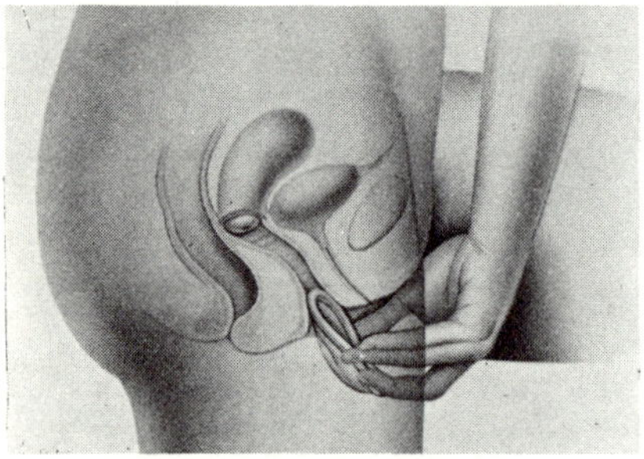

(b) Insertion

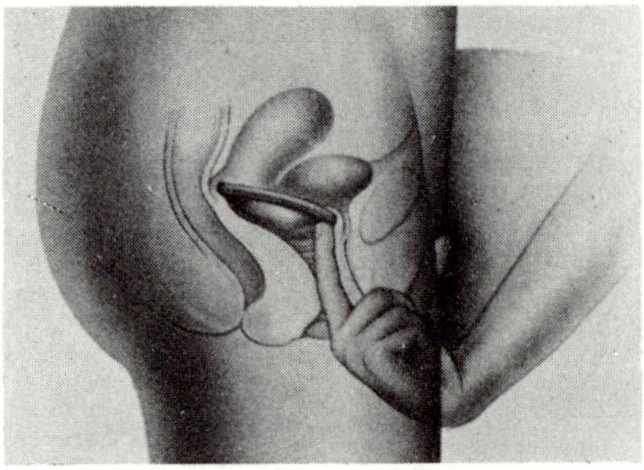

(c) Placing it correctly

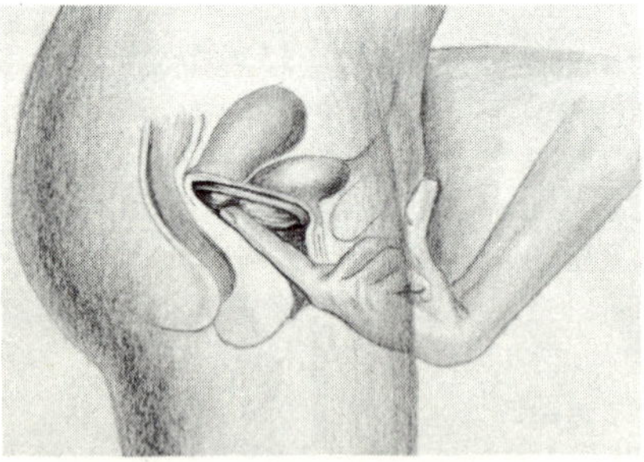

(d) Ensuring that the cervix is covered

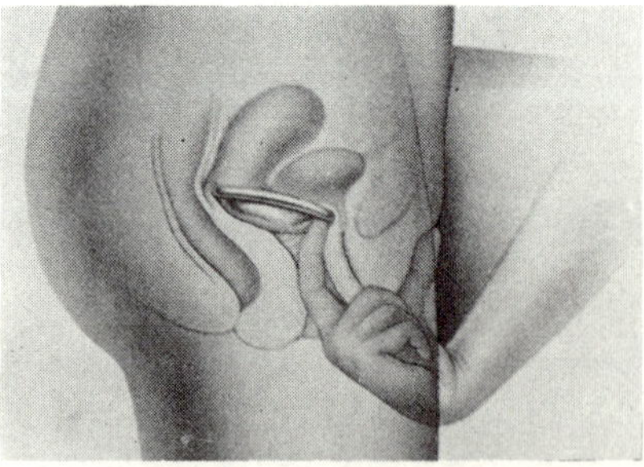

(e) Removing the diaphragm by hooking the index finger under the spring rim

FIG. 7/5. The technique used in inserting the diaphragm

If used in this way, the vaginal diaphragm is very satisfactory. Provided the correct size has been chosen, it is not apparent to either partner during sexual intercourse, and it protects against pregnancy without causing any side-effects. It requires a certain intelligence to use, as unless it is inserted properly, it may fail to cover the cervix. For this reason, after inserting the diaphragm, the woman should put a finger inside her vagina to see if she can feel the cervix through the rubber. The cervix feels like the tip of the nose. If she cannot feel the cervix through the rubber, the diaphragm is probably incorrectly placed. In fact, however, once a woman is confident about introducing a vaginal diaphragm, the method is found to be very easy. The pregnancy rate is about 9 per 100 woman years.

ORAL CONTRACEPTIVES: The ineffectiveness of coitus interruptus, the abnormal sexual restraints required by the rhythm method, and the need for reasonable privacy and manual dexterity that is demanded of vaginal diaphragm users, have meant that conception control in the first half of this century was fairly ineffective, particularly amongst those women needing it most. The better educated, richer women solved their problem, and the size of their families fell to an average of two children. The least-educated, the poor, the needy, the 'under-privileged' either resorted to induced abortion, or failed to control the size of their families, with the result that relatively more children were born to women least well able to care for them.

The whole picture has changed, at least in the affluent societies, since 1957–the 'Year of the Pill'. It had been known for some time that small doses of oestrogen given from the end of menstruation would prevent ovulation occurring. Unfortunately, the menstrual period which followed was prolonged, with many days of 'spotting' and dribbling of blood. Obviously this was intolerable for women. It was also known that if expensive injections of progesterone–the second sex hormone–were given daily for the last 6 days on which oestrogen was also given, the period would be fairly normal. Unfortunately, the method needed daily injections for 6 days each month, and women did not think much of that idea.

In the early 1950s, research workers had been trying to find a plant which would provide a substitute for progesterone, as this could only be obtained from animals, and was only effective if given by injection. One plant which seemed hopeful was a particular

Mexican yam, which after exhaustive investigation proved to yield a substance which had progesterone-like actions, and was called a 'gestagen' for that reason. This drug had the advantage that it was effective when taken by mouth. Dr. Pincus, an American scientist, set out to investigate if various combinations of oestrogens and the new gestagen would stop ovulation in animals. He found they would, and between 1955 and 1957 he conducted trials on human volunteers. Once again, the drugs used in combination proved effective in stopping ovulation, and did so without affecting the menstrual periods. It was evident that here was a method of contraception which should be of great value to women. The mixture of the drugs was called an 'oral contraceptive'; later this was shortened by general usage to 'the Pill', although by that time there were many pills of different combinations of the two drugs. 'The Pill' has several advantages. It is easy to take, no privacy is needed to take it, it is nearly 100 per cent effective, and when taken for 21 or 22 days each month it protects the woman against pregnancy no matter when sexual intercourse takes place during the cycle.

Oral contraceptives today: Since those early days, many new forms of 'the Pill' have come onto the market, and today three main kinds are available. The original Pill consisted of a mixture of oestrogen and gestagen, and was called the Combined Pill. The Combined Pill was taken for 21 days, starting on day 5 of the menstrual cycle. This may appear a little confusing, but really is not. The day that menstruation *starts* is day 1, so that the Pill was first taken from the fifth day after the start of menstruation. As time has passed, it has been found that the amount of the two sex hormones in the Combined Pill could be reduced considerably without reducing its efficiency in preventing pregnancy, so that today's Combined Pills are low-dosage pills.

One group of researchers felt that it might be better if in the first half of the cycle only oestrogen, or perhaps oestrogen with a tiny amount of gestagen, was given, and in the second half the Combined Pill was used. It was hoped that this would reduce the amount of the drugs needed still further, and reduce the side-effects of the drugs which were annoying to some women. Also, because some women could not count, a pack was made up with the oral contraceptive pills which were taken for 21 days and then 7 sugar pills, one of which was taken each day from day 22 and through menstruation.

This meant that the woman took a pill a day, and led to the slogan 'a pill a day keeps pregnancy at bay'. The pills used in this method were called Sequential or Serial Pills. They have been found to be a little less effective in preventing pregnancy than the Combined Pill, but still have a Pregnancy Index of 2 per 100 woman years, compared with the Combined Pill rate of less than 1 per 100 woman years.

Recently a third kind of oral contraceptive pill has been introduced. This consists of the gestagen only, and is taken each day continuously. The idea was that if oestrogen was left out, the side-effects due to oestrogen would stop, and this would be an advantage. The Gestagen Pill, as it is called, is only fairly successful, as about one woman in five bleeds at irregular intervals instead of having regular periods, and the Pregnancy Index is about 6 per 100 woman years, more than double that of the Sequential Pill. Nevertheless, the Gestagen Pill has a place in oral contraception.

Side-effects of oral contraceptives: The side-effects of the pills are due to the hormones which they contain, working on the body either alone or in combination. The most common complaint, which occurs in about one woman in five in the first cycle, is nausea. Usually by the third menstrual cycle this side-effect has gone, as the woman's body has 'adjusted' to the hormones. A few women develop an increased amount of clear vaginal discharge in each cycle whilst taking the Pill. This is worse halfway between the periods, but unless it causes itchiness, it does not require any treatment. Some women who take the Pill notice that their breasts are uncomfortable, and that they have put on a few pounds in weight just before a period, but the weight disappears after the period. These symptoms, and the occasional occurrence of headaches, are due to the retention of water in the tissues of the body. These side-effects, and all the others mentioned, are due to the oestrogen part of the Pill, and so do not occur with the Continuous Gestagen Pill. However, oestrogen has some beneficial side-effects. Women who have painful periods find that dysmenorrhoea is relieved when they take the Pill, and women who have acne find that their complexion improves.

It is usual for the amount of blood lost during the menstrual period to be reduced when taking the Pill, but some women have spotting of blood, or a slightly heavier blood loss called 'breakthrough bleeding' during a cycle when the Pill is taken. These effects are due to the gestagen. If a woman does have 'spotting' or 'breakthrough bleeding', she should take an extra pill for a couple of days until it ceases. One other effect due to the gestagen needs mentioning. If the Pill is taken over several months, some women gain in weight. This weight gain does not appear before and disappear after a menstrual period–it is there all the time–and is due to fat being deposited in the tissues. Usually the gain is about 3 to 5 lb., but some women put on a lot more.

A few women, luckily very few, develop side-effects due to both the oestrogen and the gestagen. The side-effects vary from month to month, and in some months may be absent, but when present are annoying. They are mood changes, the woman becoming irritable, unduly tired, sometimes unusually aggressive, and occasionally suffering a reduction in sexual desire.

The most written-about side-effect has been left to the last. This is the increased risk of a clot forming in a vein, and it is probably due to the oestrogen part of the Pill. But the matter should be put in perspective. Only one woman in every 2,000 taking the Pill will develop a blood clot in a vein, and if she were pregnant each year, she has twice the chance of developing a clot.

Women who should not take the Pill: Certain women should not use oral contraceptives, as they have conditions which will make the side-effects quite severe. These are women who have previously had a clot in a *deep* vein; women who have liver disease; women who have a very high blood pressure; women who have severe migraine; and women who have certain blood disorders. For these women, there are other more suitable methods of contraception.

Before the Pill is prescribed: Because of the side-effects, no woman should be prescribed the Pill without having been examined by a doctor who can make sure that she has none of the diseases mentioned. He will also examine her breasts and do a pelvic examination, to make sure that her genital organs are normal. If she has not had a 'cervical smear' ('Pap Test') for cancer of the cervix done in the preceding year, the doctor will also make this test.

The first month in which the Pill is taken needs care, as pregnancies have occurred in this cycle. Either the patient should avoid sexual intercourse during the first half of the month, or else she or her husband should use some other form of contraceptive for this particular cycle.

Possible long-term effects of the Pill: Women have taken the Pill for nearly 10 years now, and no dangerous long-term effects have been found. There is no evidence that taking the Pill impairs the fertility of a woman when she stops and decides to have a baby. In fact her fertility may be increased for a short while. A point to note here is that some women find that their first menstrual period after stopping the Pill is delayed for 2 or 3 weeks. This may make the diagnosis of pregnancy more difficult, but a doctor can usually tell. Very occasionally, too, a woman's periods cease when she stops the Pill. There is no harm from this, as they usually start again after a few months, and can always be started by giving a special drug which is taken by mouth. Finally, from studies made since the Pill was introduced, no evidence has appeared that the Pill causes cancer.

The Pill after childbirth: It is unlikely that ovulation will occur for at least 20 weeks if the mother is breast-feeding her baby, although it may. For this reason, many women do not want to take a chance and decide to take the Pill. There is no need for them to do this before the postnatal visit, and at that time the doctor can easily prescribe the Pill. There is some evidence that the continuous Gestagen Pill is the most suitable, but provided that the milk is flowing freely, any of the oral contraceptives can be used without reducing its flow.

The future: Although the oral contraceptives have been said to have emancipated womankind from constant childbearing, they are not without drawbacks. They are unsuitable for some women, or have been used and given up by others for a variety of reasons, usually because of side-effects or because another pregnancy was planned. Research continues to find oral contraceptives with fewer side-effects, which are cheaper but as efficient.

THE INTRAUTERINE CONTRACEPTIVE DEVICE: The Pill is fairly expensive; not too expensive for women in affluent countries, but far too expensive for the great masses of women who live in the developing lands of the world. Moreover, the Pill needs to be taken each day for 21 days of the month, and women who never use a calendar may well forget. Because of this, researchers sought other methods which were cheap and effective. One of these is the intrauterine contraceptive device.

There is nothing new about the intrauterine contraceptive device. Arab camel drivers in Biblical times used the method. They used to introduce a round stone, the size of a pea, into the uterus of their female camels, which then repulsed the advances of the male camels, and worked harder! In the 1920s, a German gynaecologist used a silver or gold device which he introduced into the womb. Unfortunately it caused many complications and was abandoned by most doctors as unsafe.

A revival of interest in this form of contraception occurred after the discovery of polythene. Polythene is a plastic, which easily regains its shape after stretching, is not irritating to the tissues, and can be made free from germs quite easily. Because of the urgent need for some cheap form of contraceptive device, various shapes of polythene were devised to see if they would prevent pregnancy when inserted into the uterus of a woman. From all of these shapes the Loop and the Spiral have been developed, and of the two, the Loop seems the more effective (Fig. **7/6**).

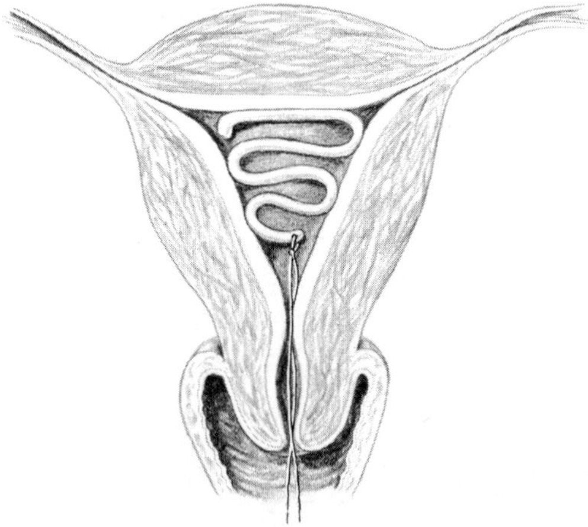

FIG. 7/6. The intrauterine contraceptive device

If a woman decides that she will use the Loop for contraceptive purposes, she must first be examined by a doctor to make sure that her uterus is normal and that she has no infection in her pelvis. At the same time the doctor takes a 'Pap smear' from the cervix. The Loop is straightened by inserting it into a narrow curved tube. The tip of this tube is then pushed gently through the cervical canal so that its tip lies just inside the lower part of the uterus. With a plunger, the Loop is now pushed into the womb, where it regains its shape. The operation is complete.

After the Loop is inserted, the patient may have a few colicky pains during the first month, and she may have 'spotting' or bleeding, but these symptoms usually settle down. More serious, the uterus may expel the Loop, and this occurs in 1 patient in every 10. It is for this reason that the Loop has a tail made of two soft nylon threads. Each evening the patient should put a finger high in her vagina to make sure that the threads can be felt. If she cannot feel the threads, she should see her doctor.

The side-effects of expulsion of the Loop, bleeding episodes and pain, make this method unsatisfactory for about 1 woman in 5. These women therefore change to another method of contraception during the first year after insertion of the Loop. Unfortunately, too, it is not as efficient as oral contraception, having a Pregnancy Rate of 5 per 100 woman years.

However, in the developing countries, and especially in India, the Loop has many advantages. It is very cheap, and once it has been put in the uterus, can be left for several years, unless the patient expels it or wishes to have it removed. Therefore one doctor can fit many patients, and once fitted, the patient needs to take no further action to avoid pregnancy. She does not need privacy or intelligence, as she would if she used the vaginal diaphragm; nor does she need money and some intelligence, as she would if she decided to use oral contraceptives. In India over 15 million women have been fitted with the Loop.

Table 7/1

Use-effectiveness of various contraceptives
(Pregnancies per 1200 months of exposure)

No contraception	180
Condom	15
Withdrawal	35
Rhythm method	30
Vaginal douching	45
Vaginal jellies or creams	40
Vaginal diaphragm + spermicidal jelly	9
Intrauterine contraceptive device	5
Oral contraceptives:	
Combined	0.25
Sequential	2
Continuous gestagen	6

TUBAL LIGATION: If a patient has had all the children she and her husband will ever want, she can avoid further pregnancies by an operation. This operation is done under an anaesthetic by making a small cut in the abdominal wall, and then by cutting out a wedge from each oviduct, or Fallopian tube (Fig. 7/7). By doing this, the

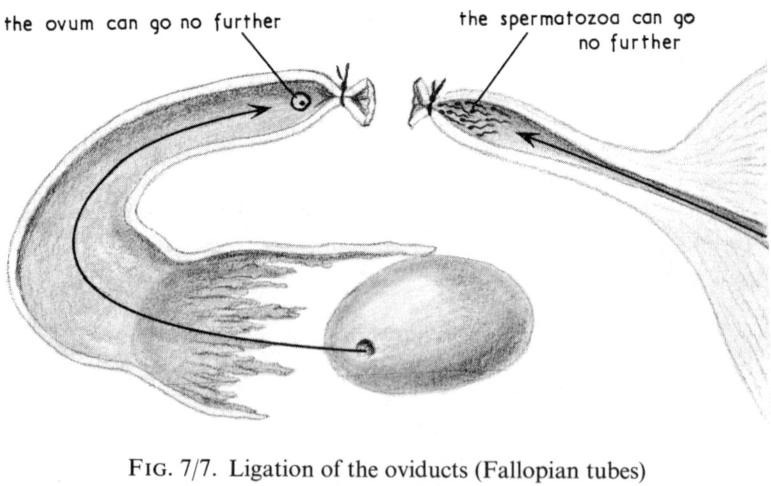

FIG. 7/7. Ligation of the oviducts (Fallopian tubes)

spermatozoa are prevented from reaching the ovum, and no other form of contraception is required. The operation is 100 per cent effective, and once done cannot easily be undone, so that the woman is permanently sterile. This is why tubal ligation can only be performed with the agreement of both husband and wife, and in the knowledge that it is the 'final solution' to fertility.

Strange myths surround the operation. They are that after tubal ligation (or 'sterilization' as it is sometimes wrongly called), the woman loses her sexual urge, her periods stop, she gets fat, and after a few years the oviducts open up and pregnancy becomes possible once more. These 'folk-tales' are all untrue. After tubal ligation the woman notices no difference in her sex urge, her periods continue as normal, she does not get fat (unless she overeats), and the operation provides permanent protection against pregnancy.

Contraception after the age of 40

It is not certain for how many years a woman past the age of 40 should use contraceptives in order to avoid any possibility of pregnancy. Ovulation occurs less frequently after the age of 40, and rarely after the age of 47. At the moment, then, it would seem wise for her to continue with contraception until the age of 50. If she is taking the Pill she will, of course, continue to bleed each month, and will not know when she has reached the natural menopause, or 'change of life'.

CHAPTER 8

A slight touch of pregnancy

Most women have a pretty good idea that they may be pregnant before they consult a doctor to confirm their suspicions. For most, the confirmation is an occasion for joy; for some an occasion for anxiety and sorrow. A few women, desperately wishing to become pregnant, can mimic many of the signs of pregnancy, and believe themselves to be pregnant when in fact they are not. Even after the doctor has told the patient that she is not pregnant, she refuses to believe him. These patients have a 'phantom pregnancy', and require sympathetic psychiatric attention.

THE SYMPTOMS OF EARLY PREGNANCY

Amenorrhoea

The first symptom of pregnancy is usually that the menstrual period fails to occur on the expected date. If a woman has regular periods and has had the chance of becoming pregnant, the absence of menstruation (or amenorrhoea) suggests that she is pregnant. But a woman who has regular periods should wait at least 10 days before consulting a doctor, as before this time he will not be able to tell if she is pregnant. If her periods are not regular, amenorrhoea is less helpful in making a diagnosis of pregnancy.

Pregnancy is the most usual cause of amenorrhoea in women aged 16 to 40, but it is not the only cause. Menstruation may be delayed or suppressed by the emotions, in certain illnesses and when certain drugs are taken. Emotional stress is the most usual cause of amenorrhoea, apart from pregnancy, in a woman who has previously menstruated normally. The emotions act on the part of the brain which controls the release of hormones. Fear of an unwanted pregnancy; a fight with a loved one; a new and difficult job; or a journey, all can cause amenorrhoea.

Breast changes

Many women experience breast fullness and discomfort just prior to their menstrual period. If pregnancy occurs, these symptoms persist and are increased. The breasts become fuller, firmer and more tender. Occasionally they throb and the nipples tingle. The degree of these symptoms is quite variable, but as pregnancy advances the fullness of the breasts increases, and the nipples become larger and darker. The area around the nipple, which is called the areola, also becomes larger, darker and rather swollen. In this area there are tiny openings to milk ducts and minute glands. In pregnancy the minute milk glands and ducts enlarge to form small protuberances or follicles – which are named Montgomery's follicles after an Irish obstetrician who first described them. These are rarely noticeable until the pregnancy is 8 weeks advanced.

The changes in the breasts are caused by the female sex hormones oestrogen and progesterone produced by the placenta. These hormones cause growth of the ducts and milk sacs of the breast, and lead to fat being deposited around the milk apparatus to cushion it. The tingling and throbbing occasionally felt is due to the increased flow of blood through the blood vessels which supply the breasts.

Nausea and vomiting

In about half of pregnant women some degree of nausea or vomiting occurs. Usually this is quite mild, and occurs in the morning. Occasionally, however, it is more severe, and vomiting may occur at any time of the day. When this occurs, it usually starts about 2 weeks after the first missed period, and lasts for about 6 to 8 weeks. The cause of the nausea is not known, but it seems probable that it is due to the increases in the amount of sex hormones produced in pregnancy. It usually goes by the 12th week of pregnancy as the body adjusts to the changes.

Bladder 'irritability'

In early pregnancy the kidneys function over-efficiently, and the bladder fills with urine more quickly. This leads to frequency of urination, which is an early symptom of pregnancy.

WHAT THE DOCTOR LOOKS FOR

The patient visiting her doctor in early pregnancy will be asked about the symptoms just mentioned, and will then be examined. As will be described in the chapter on antenatal care, the examination includes a careful assessment of the patient's general health, in which the heart is listened to, the breasts are examined, the abdomen is palpated, and an 'internal', or pelvic, examination is performed. This examination need not be feared, as it is quite painless. The patient lies on her back with her legs bent and her knees apart. She breathes slowly and relaxes all her muscles. The doctor first examines her vulva and then gently introduces a small instrument, called a speculum, into the vagina so that he may look at the cervix. Many doctors take this opportunity to take a sample of the cells which cover the cervix, so that these may be examined in the laboratory. This is called the 'Pap smear' test, after Dr. Papanicolaou who first described it. Abnormal cells are found in about 1 sample in every 200 examined. These patients have to be investigated further in case the abnormal cells indicate a very early cancer of the cervix. The doctor then removes the speculum and putting on a plastic glove, inserts two fingers into the vagina. With his other hand he presses gently on the abdomen just below the umbilicus (Fig. **8/1**). In this way he can feel the shape of the uterus and tell if it is enlarged, as would be expected in pregnancy, or if there are any other swellings which may require treatment. The pelvic examination is most informative when made between the 6th and 10th week of pregnancy.

TESTS FOR PREGNANCY

Immunological tests

After the general and pelvic examinations, the doctor may still be unsure if the patient is pregnant, so he may make a test on the

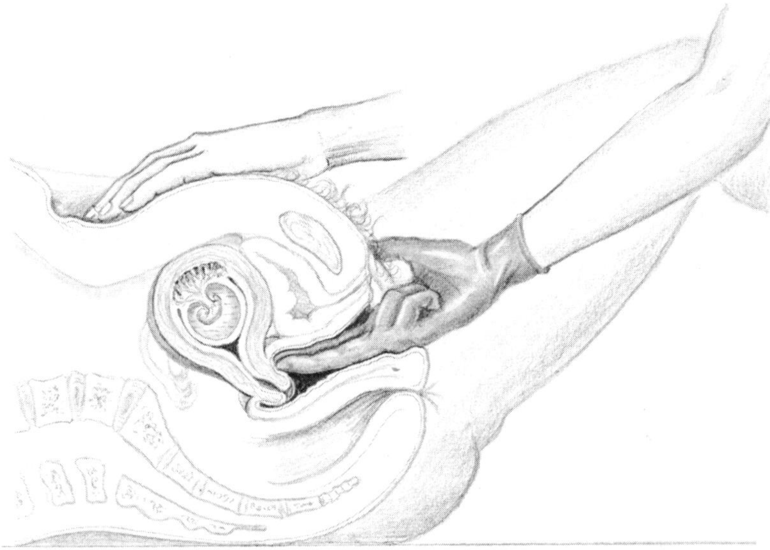

FIG. 8/1. The diagnosis of early pregnancy

patient's urine. This test depends on the fact that within 40 days of the last menstrual period, a large amount of a special hormone called HCG, made by the placenta, circulates in the blood. This hormone is then excreted in the urine and can be measured by a simple test. A drop of a substance which neutralizes HCG (anti-HCG) is put on a glass slide, and a drop of the patient's urine is added. The two drops are mixed, and after a minute two drops of a milky substance made of latex rubber particles covered with HCG are added. If the patient is not pregnant, the anti-HCG substance will fix onto the HCG covering the latex, and they will clump together to form 'curds' in the milky substance. However, if the patient is pregnant, all the anti-HCG will have joined with the HCG in the urine, and none will be left over to combine with the HCG on the latex particles. Because of this, the particles will not clump and the milky solution has no curds when examined. The test takes two minutes to perform, and is 95 per cent accurate after the 40th day of pregnancy. It is called the 'agglutination-inhibition test for pregnancy' (Fig. **8/2**).

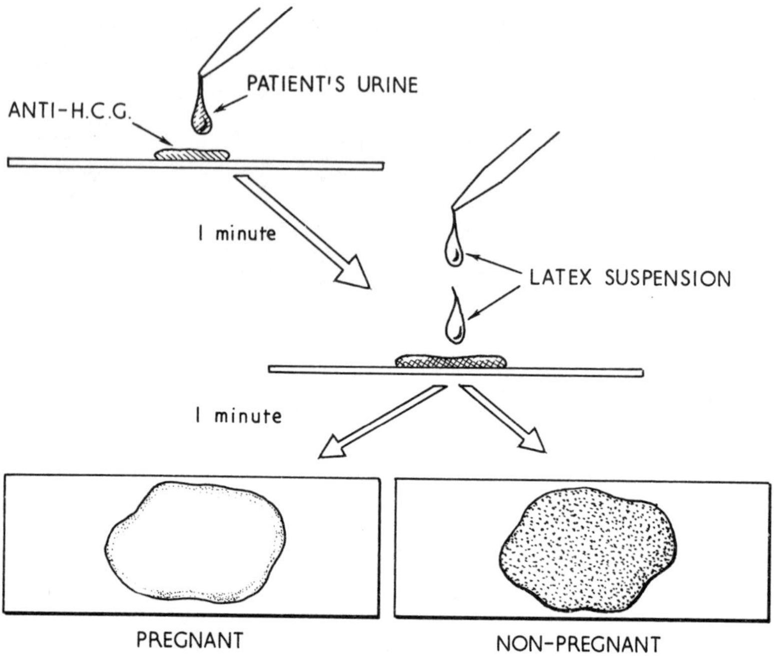

FIG. 8/2. How pregnancy is diagnosed by a 'slide test'

Ultrasound

An even more exciting development is a machine which uses 'radar' to detect if a pregnancy is present. The machine uses ultrasound (that is, sound waves of a very high frequency). The sound waves 'echo' off different tissues and can be translated into a picture. The machine has many uses in obstetrics, as well as diagnosing early pregnancy. In early pregnancy it can detect an ectopic pregnancy, in which the embryo is in the oviduct, not the uterus. In late pregnancy it can detect the position of the baby, the presence of twins, the position of the placenta, and by taking readings at intervals, it is possible to determine the speed of growth of the baby. The machine is expensive, but as time passes more and more hospitals will be able to offer this diagnostic service to patients.

THE SYMPTOMS AND SIGNS OF LATER PREGNANCY

As the uterus grows, its size becomes obvious, however much a woman may desire her dressmaker to hide it! After the 16th week of pregnancy, other symptoms and signs also indicate pregnancy, although by this time it should be pretty obvious to any intelligent woman that she is pregnant.

'Quickening'

At about 18 to 20 weeks in first pregnancies and two weeks earlier in subsequent pregnancies, the first faint fluttering movements of the baby are felt. This is called 'quickening' because once it was believed that the baby only became alive at this time. It is reflected by the Biblical reference to the 'quick and the dead'.

Movements of the fetus become stronger and more frequent as pregnancy advances, and the mother may notice that her baby has periods of activity and periods of rest. In the rest periods, it probably sleeps. Provided the periods of activity and rest coincide with the same periods in the mother, all is well; but some babies seem to take a perverse delight in having their active periods at night, to the annoyance of the mother! If the movements are very active, lumps appear and disappear on the uterus and are noticed by the mother. They are caused by the baby's limbs stretching the muscles of the uterus. Many babies are less active, and sometimes a day or more passes without movements being felt. This does not mean that the baby is dead, but if the patient feels no movements for a longer period, she should consult her doctor, who will listen for fetal heart sounds. Recently a machine, called a Fetal Heart Detector, has been developed which relies on the 'doppler principle' of sound waves. This machine can detect the baby's heart beats as early as the 12th week of pregnancy, and is nearly 100 per cent accurate after the 16th week.

Frequency of urination

Frequency of urination, which was a symptom of early pregnancy, ceases after the 12th week, to reappear in the last weeks of pregnancy. In late pregnancy the symptom is due to the pressure of the baby's head on the bladder, and can be quite disturbing, especially at night.

WHAT THE DOCTOR FINDS IN LATE PREGNANCY

The growth of the uterus

To some extent the doctor can tell how much the pregnancy has advanced by noting the height of the top of the uterus in the patient's abdomen (Fig. **8/3**). The method is not very accurate, and various

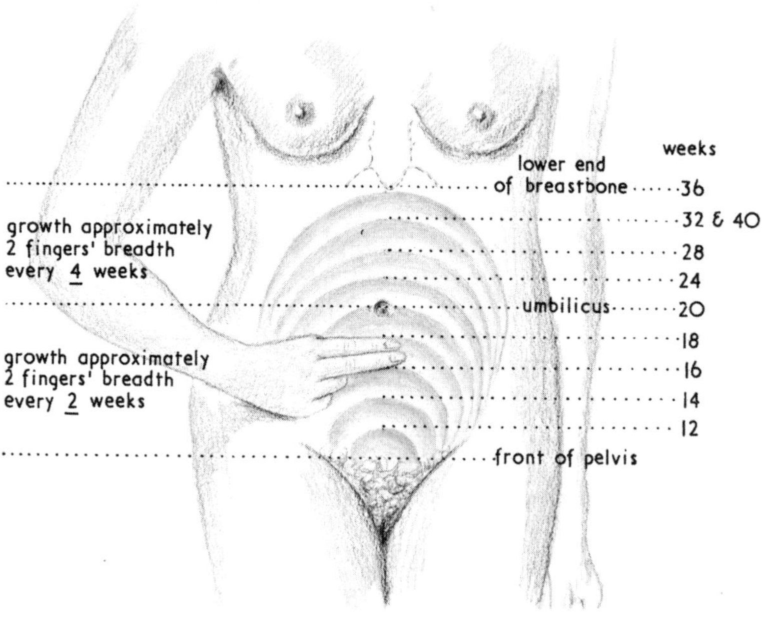

FIG. 8/3. The growth of the uterus in pregnancy

factors such as tenseness of the abdomen or obesity can lead to false readings. At the same time, the doctor gently runs his fingers over the uterus to determine the position of the baby. He should always tell the patient where her baby is lying, outlining the position for her. He usually listens for the baby's heart sounds, but if the patient is feeling the 'movements' of the baby, this is not really necessary.

The growing uterus stretches the patient's abdominal skin, and by the 20th week it will be obvious that she is pregnant. From this time on small pinkish streaks, about $1\frac{1}{2}$ in. long, appear over the lower abdomen, especially in the flanks. These 'streaks of pregnancy' are due to small breaks in the lower layer of the skin which is less well able to stretch. They also sometimes appear on the thighs. After the birth of the baby, the colour fades to silvery-white, but remains permanently. There is no known way to prevent them, although some women believe that massage of the skin with olive oil helps.

In dark-haired women, another change may be found. This is a brownish pigmented line stretching in the midline from the umbilicus to the pubic bone. It is of no consequence, and fades after delivery, almost disappearing in time.

X-rays

Occasionally the doctor has to make use of X-ray examinations to clear up an obscure point. Because X-rays have a slight potential danger if overused, the modern tendency is to use them only when really necessary. For example, the doctor may be unable to decide whether the baby is lying as a breech, or if there are twins present. In these cases an X-ray may be necessary. In other cases the patient may have felt no movements of the baby, and the doctor fails to hear the baby's heart. If he does not have a fetal heart detector, he may suggest an X-ray examination to try to determine if the baby is alive or not. Occasionally an X-ray examination of the shape of the pelvis is required if the baby's head does not settle properly into the mother's pelvis in late pregnancy.

Mothers sometimes ask if an X-ray can be taken to determine the sex of the unborn baby. Since X-rays only show up bones, it is impossible to tell the sex of the baby in this way.

CHAPTER 9

A most wondrous growth

THE FETUS

Fertilization occurs in the outer part of the oviduct, when a single spermatozoon penetrates the 'shell' (or zona pellucida) of the egg and enters its substance. The sperm's tail is stuck in the 'shell' and drops off, leaving the sperm head free in the egg. The part of the sperm head, called the nucleus, which contains in twisted strands the information needed to make a new individual, joins with the nucleus of the egg, and they fuse. The first step towards a new individual, who will take half of its characteristics from its father and half from its mother, has been taken. Inside the zona pellucida, the fertilized egg with its fused nucleus divides into 2 identical cells, then into 4 cells, then into 8 cells, then into 16 cells, and again until it looks like a mulberry made up of 64 cells. These divisions take place during the 3 days that it takes the fertilized egg to gently move along the oviduct to reach the cavity of the uterus. Inside its cavity, the fertilized egg develops further, fluid appearing amongst the mulberry cells, and eventually splitting them into two parts: an outer shell of cells, and a collection of cells at one side. The outer cells will form the placenta; the inner mass will form the embryo. Quite soon after this, on the same or the next day, the zona pellucida dissolves and the fertilized egg, now called a blastocyst, plants itself into the juicy, soft lining of the womb (Fig. **9/1**). Nine days after fertilization the blastocyst has burrowed deeply into the lining of the womb and has grown to the size of a pin-head. Four days later, at the time the menstrual period is expected, it has enlarged to be just visible to the naked eye. From now on the growth of the embryo and the placenta proceeds apace. From the very earliest time, a fluid-filled space develops around the embryo. This space is lined with a thin, glistening membrane, and this in turn is surrounded by a thicker membrane.

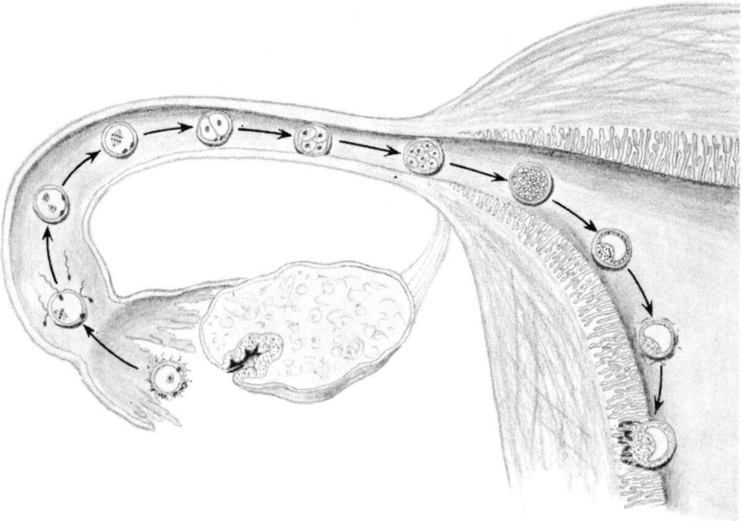

FIG. 9/1. The beginning of pregnancy
The diagram shows fertilization of the egg in the oviduct, and its development as it journeys through the oviduct to reach the uterus and implant

The membranes with the contained water are called the amniotic sac, or the bag of waters. By the 36th week of pregnancy, 1,000 ml. ($1\frac{3}{4}$ pints) of water surround the fetus. The fetus (until the 8th week of pregnancy, it is called the embryo) is able to move about freely within the amniotic sac, but it is prevented from being injured should the expectant mother fall, as the water absorbs all the shock.

Within two days of implantation, the outer cells of the blastocyst are sprouting in finger-like projections all round the sphere of the egg. Quite quickly most of them die, and only the disc of cells lying deep in the lining of the uterus continue to grow. This disc forms the placenta, through which the fetus obtains all its nourishment. The placenta is connected to the fetus by the umbilical cord. At first the umbilical cord reaches from the placenta and joins the embryo near its tail, as can be seen in Fig. **9/2**, but quite soon the tail curls round and the umbilical cord joins the fetus in the centre of its abdomen, at the place which after birth is the navel, or umbilicus. This is shown in Fig. **9/3**. In many ways the placenta and the fetus work together, which is understandable as they form from the same fertilized egg. The placenta acts as the lung, the liver and the kidney of the fetus. Oxygen for its energy needs is transferred from the mother's bloodstream, where it is carried by the red blood cells, to the blood in the fetus. Carbon dioxide, and other waste products of energy production, are transferred from the fetus to the mother's blood. This reduces the work which the fetal liver and kidney have to perform.

The fetus and the placenta work together to produce various hormones, which are so important in maintaining the pregnancy.

All these activities take place through the cells which form the placenta, and at all times the mother's blood and the blood of the fetus are completely separated. The two bloods never mix. The mother's blood bathes the placental cells, which permits them to take oxygen and nourishment from it, and to transfer them across the placenta into the network of tiny blood vessels on the fetal side of the placenta. These tiny vessels join together to form three big blood vessels, which pass along the umbilical cord to join up with the blood vessels inside the fetus. The umbilical cord is in fact a tube composed of a kind of thick jelly, through which the three vessels (two arteries and a vein) pass to link the fetus with the placenta.

It is easier to understand the further growth of the fetus and placenta by describing it at intervals: first at 6 weeks, then at 8 weeks, and then every 4 weeks to 40 weeks. In this description, the period is calculated from the first day of the last menstrual period, so the actual age of the embryo is about 2 weeks less. The new individual is called an embryo until week 8, and a fetus thereafter. During the embryonic period, all the structures which make it a normal human are formed; and subsequent development, during the fetal period, consists of growth and development of structures already formed.

To see the embryo and fetus, you have to imagine yourself inside the dark, warm, soft womb, where it grows throughout the pregnancy enclosed in the amniotic sac.

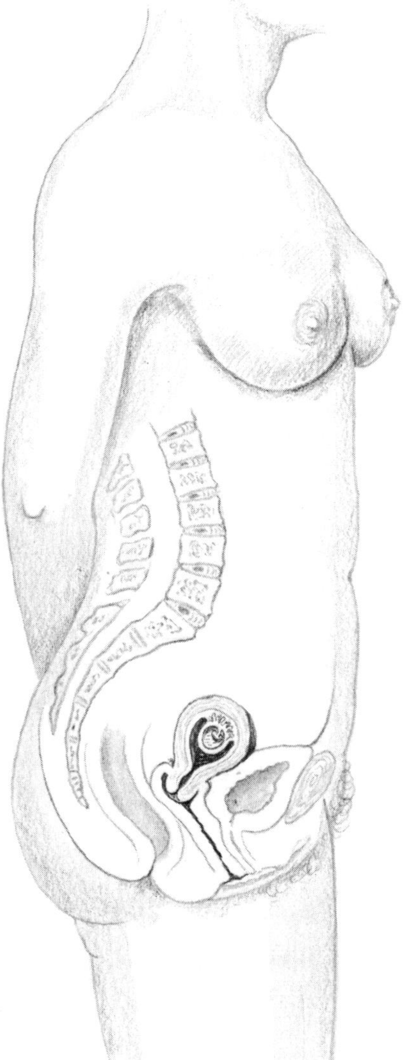

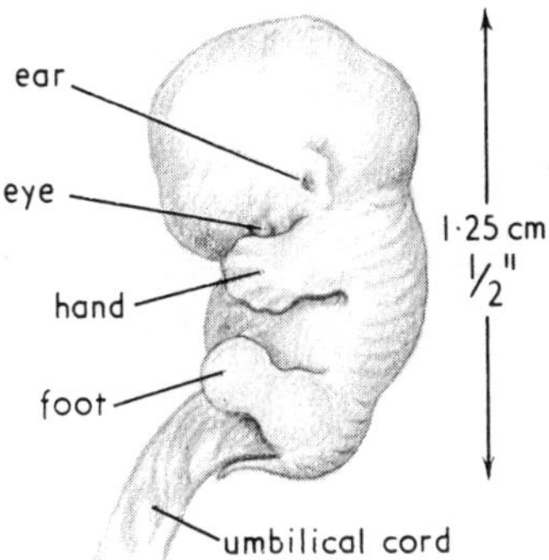

FIG. 9/2. Pregnancy at 6 weeks. The embryo is not recognizably human. It is only 28 days old, as conception occurs 14 days after the first day of the last menstrual period

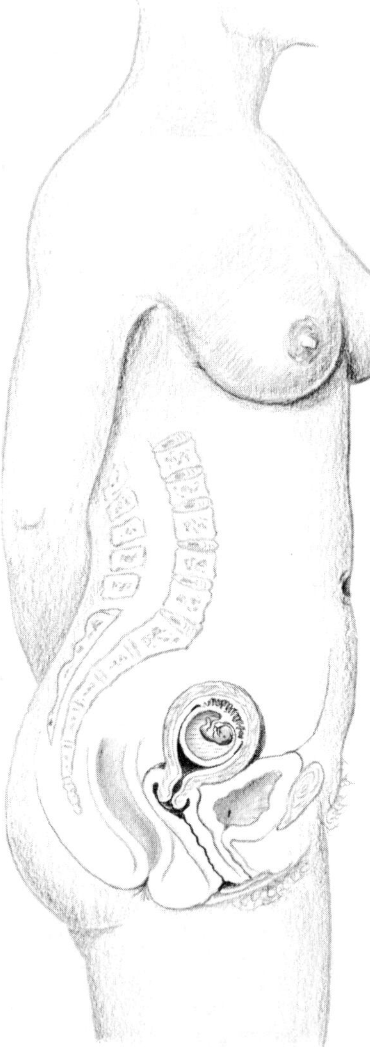

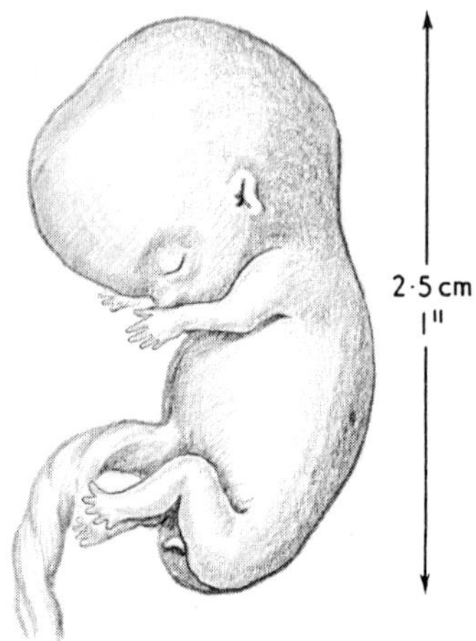

FIG. 9/3. Pregnancy at 8 weeks. The fetus is becoming more human in appearance

6 weeks
(Fig. **9/2**)

The womb has enlarged, but it is still difficult for the doctor to tell if his patient is pregnant. It has enlarged rather more than is necessary for the size of the embryo; in fact it has *anticipated* its needs. The embryo is 1.25 cm. ($\frac{1}{2}$ in.) long. Its eye socket has formed, it has a reptile-like head and a tail. Its arm and leg buds are visible, but small and spade-like in shape. The placenta is larger and weighs more than the embryo.

8 weeks
(end of the 2nd lunar month)
(Fig. **9/3**)

The womb has enlarged still more, and on a pelvic examination the doctor can tell that his patient is pregnant. Her breasts may be tender, and she may have some nausea.

The embryo is now much more like a human. It is 2.5 cm. (or 1 in.) long. The head is large compared with the body, and the external ears are forming. The limb buds have become arms and legs with tiny fingers and splayed toes. The eyes have become covered with eyelids which close across them, and remain shut until the 24th week. By now all the main organs of the body have formed, the heart beats sturdily, blood circulates through its vessels, its stomach is active and the kidneys are beginning to function. The only changes in the organs from now on will be an increase in their size and the sophistication of their function.

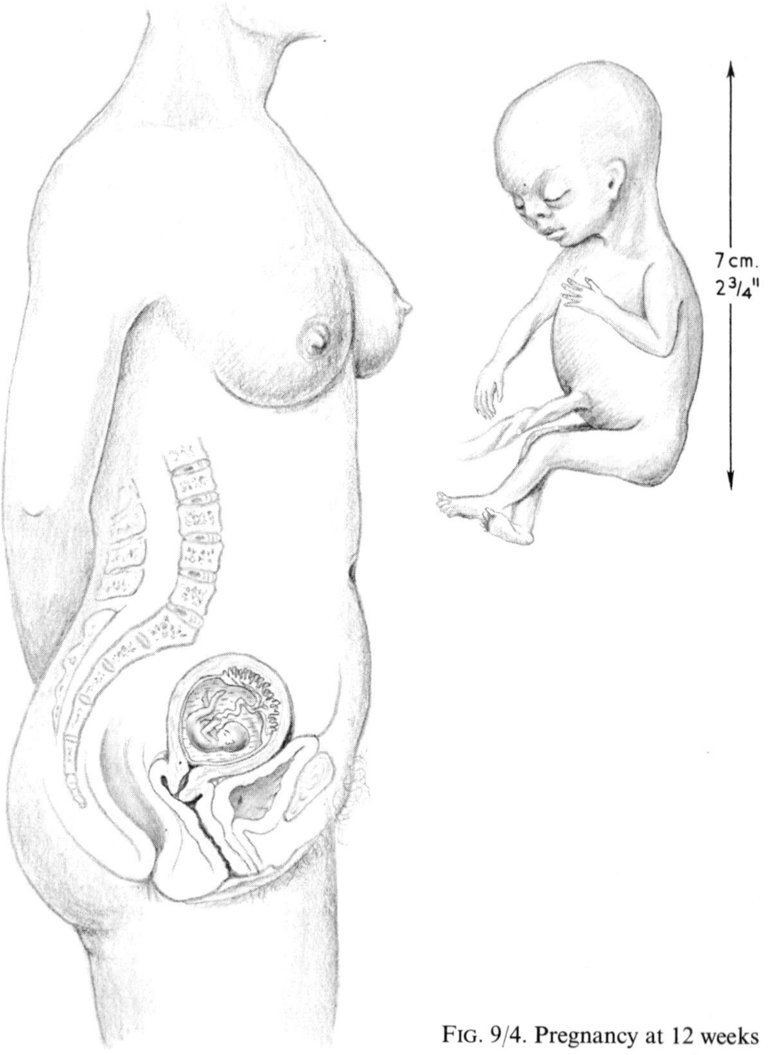

FIG. 9/4. Pregnancy at 12 weeks

12 weeks (end of the 3rd lunar month) (Fig. **9/4**)

The uterus can just be felt peeping out of the pelvis, above the symphysis. The patient is sure that she is pregnant, and the nausea is almost gone.

The fetus, as it is now called, from the Latin, meaning a 'young one', is 9 cm. ($3\frac{1}{2}$ in.) long, and weighs 14 g. ($\frac{1}{2}$ oz.). The body has grown, but the head is still over-large. Nails are appearing on its fingers and toes. The external genitals are appearing, but it is still difficult to tell its sex. By the end of this week, the mechanical movements of legs and arms have changed into movements which are far more graceful and purposeful, as the nerve and muscle co-ordination improves, although the movements are tiny. The fetus can now swallow, and begins to swallow the amniotic fluid in which it lives. At the same time, it begins to pass drops of urine into the amniotic sac. The placenta has also grown, and now weighs about six times that of the fetus.

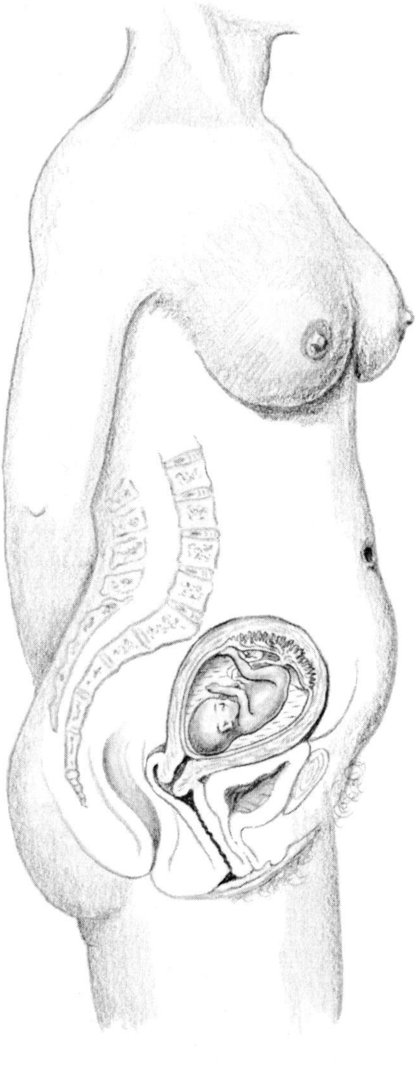

FIG. 9/5. Pregnancy at 16 weeks

16 weeks
(end of the 4th lunar month)
(Fig. **9/5**)

The uterus is easily palpable, and reaches almost halfway to the umbilicus. It is beginning to make a bulge!

The fetus is now 18 cm. (7 in.) long, and weighs 100 g (4 oz.). The head is still large for its thin body, which is bright red because the blood vessels glow through its transparent skin. Its heart is beating strongly, and its muscles are becoming active. Its sex can be distinguished. The growth of the placenta has slowed down, although its efficiency has increased, and now the weight of the placenta and the fetus are about equal.

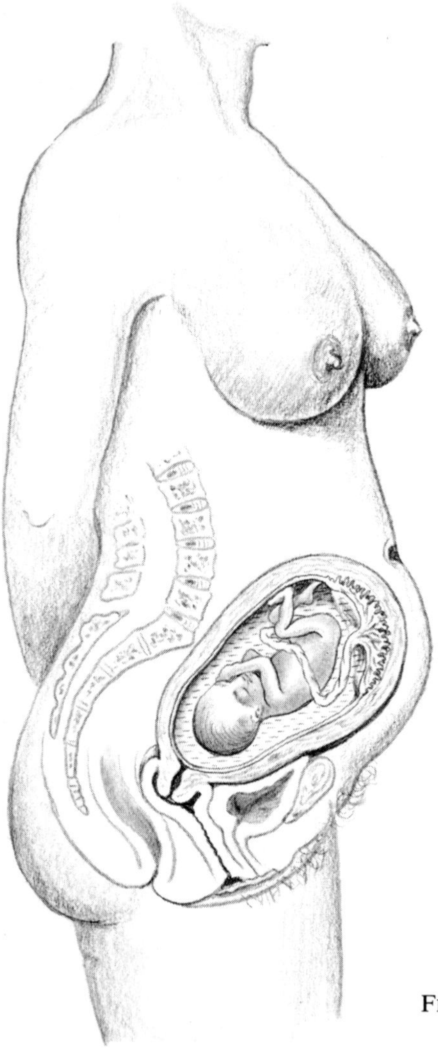

FIG. 9/6. Pregnancy at 20 weeks

20 weeks
(end of the
5th lunar month)
(Fig. **9/6**)

The uterus reaches to the level of the umbilicus and the bulge is obvious, so pregnancy can hardly be concealed. But why conceal it, the expectant mother feels so well? What is more, she has probably felt the first small 'flutters' of her baby moving in the uterus.

The fetus is now clearly human in appearance, and has 'quickened'. It is about 25 cm. (10 in.) long, and weighs about 300 g. (11 oz.). Its skin is less transparent and is covered with a fine, downy hair (called lanugo), which covers its whole body. Some hair is appearing on its head; it has developed eyebrows, but its eyelids are still completely fused. It is very active in its weightless condition within the amniotic sac. Its internal organs are becoming more mature, but as yet its lungs are insufficiently developed to cope with life outside the uterus. It is a bit like an astronaut in space! It swims weightless in its heat-controlled capsule. Its food and oxygen are conveyed to it and its waste products excreted through its lifeline–the umbilical cord. The placenta and the mother act as its life-survival pack. From this stage of pregnancy onwards, the growth of the placenta slows down, whilst that of the fetus increases, so that by 40 weeks the placenta only weighs one-fifth the weight of the baby. However, its efficiency as an exchanger for oxygen, nutrients and waste products continues to increase up to the 40th week of pregnancy.

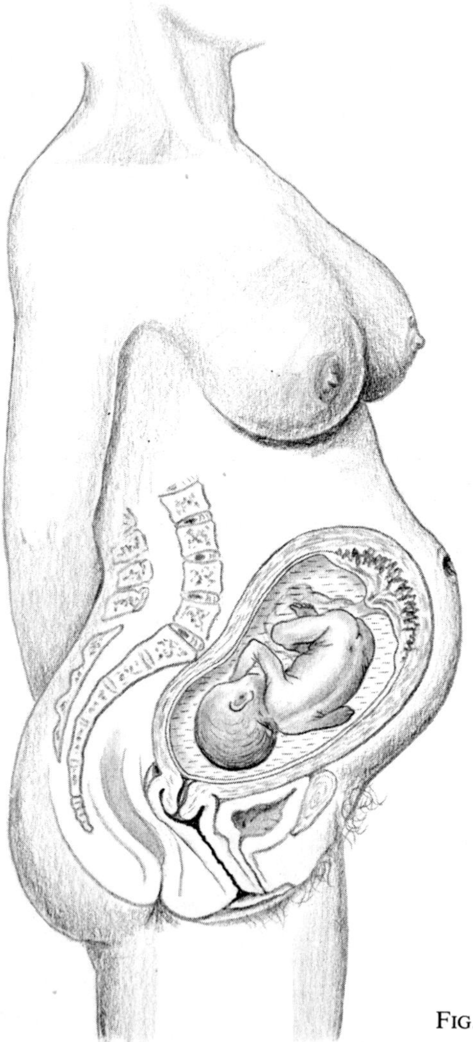

FIG. 9/7. Pregnancy at 24 weeks

24 weeks
(end of the
6th lunar month)
(Fig. **9/7**)

The expectant mother is now obviously pregnant! Her fetus measures 32 cm. (13 in.), and weighs 650 g. (1 lb. 7 oz.). Its skin is now less red, and is covered with lanugo, and wrinkled because it lacks fat. From this month on, fat will be deposited in the skin. Its eyelids have separated, but a membrane covers the pupils, which are dull. The head is comparatively large. If the fetus is born at this stage, it will attempt to breathe, but its lungs are not properly developed and it will almost certainly die soon after birth.

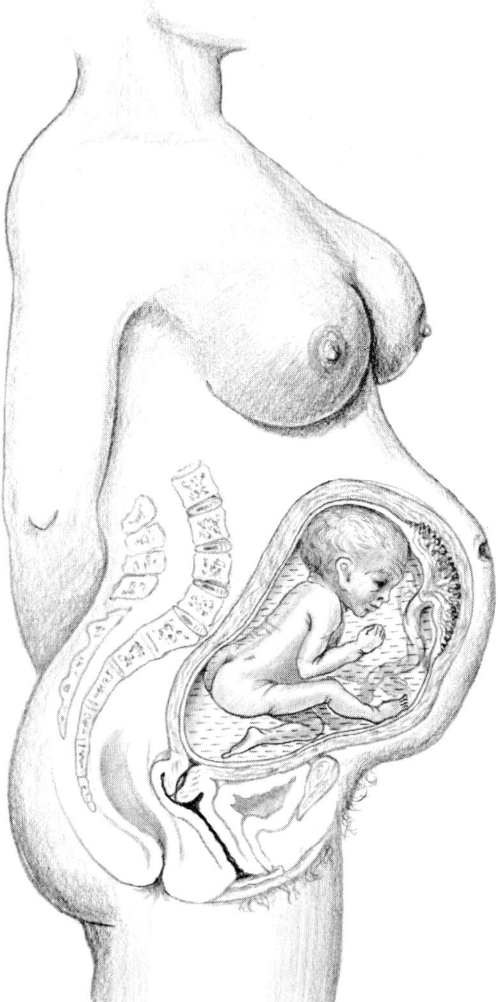

FIG. 9/8. Pregnancy at 28 weeks

28 weeks
(end of the
7th lunar month)
(Fig. **9/8**)

The uterus now reaches 4 finger-breadths above the umbilicus.

The fetus moves around vigorously within the uterus, and its heart can be heard distinctly by the doctor. Its length is 38 cm. (15 in.), and its weight 1,000 gm. (2 lb. 2 oz.). Its body is thin; its skin still reddish and covered with a protective coating of a creamy, waxy substance, called vernix caseosa, which is manufactured by small glands in the skin. It can open its eyes, and the membrane covering the pupils has gone. If born at this stage, it can now breathe (but with difficulty), cry weakly, but move its legs energetically. Usually it dies, but with good luck and careful attention in a premature unit, it may survive.

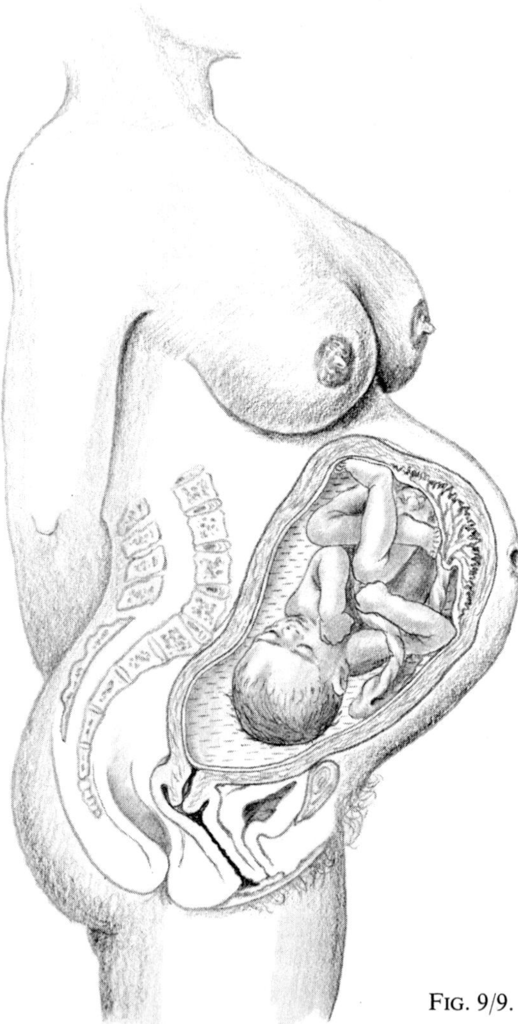

FIG. 9/9. Pregnancy at 32 weeks

A most wondrous growth

32 weeks
(end of the
8th lunar month)
(Fig. **9/9**)

The fetus is now 43 cm. (17 in.) long, and weighs about 1,800 g. (4 lb.). The skin is still reddened, rather wrinkled, but some fat is being deposited. The bones of its head are soft and flexible. Its lungs have developed and can now support life. If born at this stage, it has a good chance of surviving, provided it receives expert care.

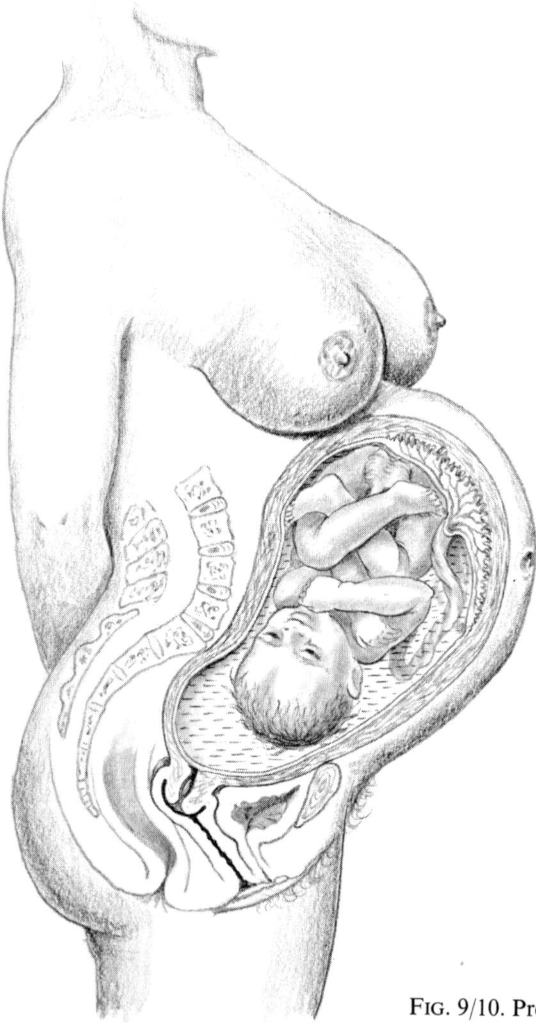

FIG. 9/10. Pregnancy at 36 weeks

36 weeks
(end of the
9th lunar month)
(Fig. **9/10**)

The uterus now reaches up to the ribcage, and may cause some discomfort. The expectant mother throws her shoulders back to keep her balance.

The fetus measures 46 cm. (18½ in.), and weighs 2,500 g. (5½ lb.). It has put on a great deal of weight, 700 g. (1½ lb.) in the preceding four weeks. This is because fat has been deposited beneath its skin and around its shoulders. It has filled out; its body has become rotund, and its face has lost its wrinkled appearance. Its finger-nails reach to the end of its fingers.

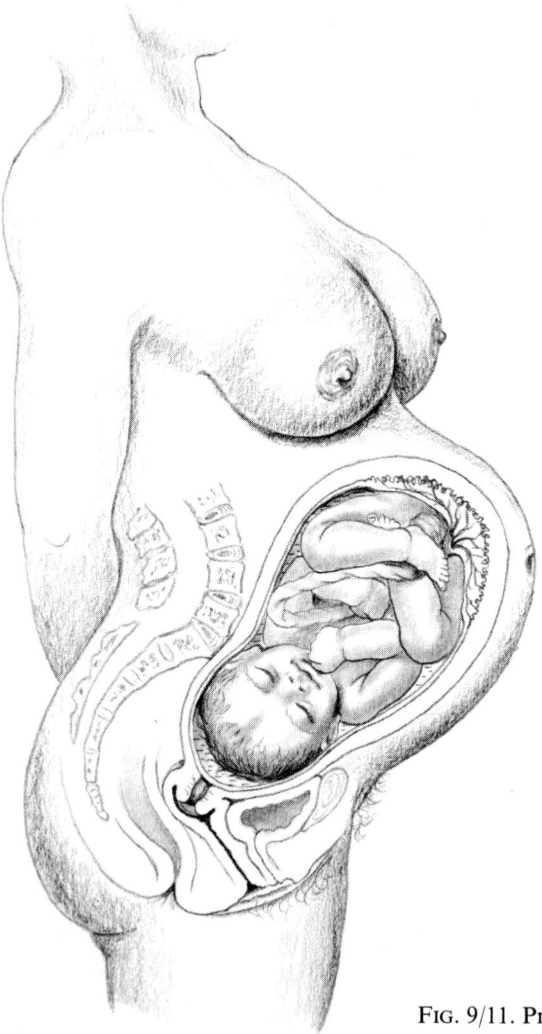

FIG. 9/11. Pregnancy at 40 weeks

40 weeks
(end of the
10th lunar month)
(Fig. **9/11**)

The pregnancy is now at its full term. The expectant mother awaits the birth of her child with some degree of impatience.

The child is 50 cm. (20 in.) long, and weighs about 3,300 g. (7 lb. 4 oz.), boys being about 100 g. (3 oz.) heavier than girls. There are very wide variations in the birth weight of the baby, and a normal, healthy, full-term child may weigh as little as 2,500 g. ($5\frac{1}{2}$ lb.) or as much as 4,500 g. (10 lb.). Occasionally the baby weighs even more. Its skin is smooth, and the lanugo which covered it has disappeared, except over the shoulders. The skin is still covered with the greasy vernix caseosa. Its head is covered with a variable amount of hair. The bones of the head are much firmer and are closer together, but the diamond-shaped soft area above the forehead and the Y-shaped area at the back of the head can still be felt. The head is now proportionate to the body, measuring about one-quarter of the body's length. The eyes are open, but usually a dull, slate colour–the permanent colour appears later. The ears stand out from the head, and the nose is well formed. The genitals are well formed, and if the infant is male, the testicles are in the scrotum.

CHANGES IN THE EXPECTANT MOTHER

Whilst the development of the embryo and fetus is progressing in the dark confines of the uterus, all the functions of the expectant mother's body are adjusting to the needs of pregnancy. The basis of all these changes is the effect of the sex hormones oestrogen and progesterone, which are manufactured by the cells of the placenta from its earliest days. The changes start very early in pregnancy, and most of them anticipate the demands that the fetus will make on its mother for oxygen, for food and to get rid of its wastes. In the early embryonic weeks, when the embryo's organs are forming at an incredible rate, the mother easily supplies the required oxygen and foods; in the later fetal weeks, when its growth is increasing even more, the fetus needs larger supplies of oxygen and nutrients for a longer period. The mother's body adjusts to these demands by quieting-down her own functions, so that nutrients (especially sugars) stay longer in her blood, and are more easily extracted by the placenta for the use of the fetus. Further energy is spared by the placidity which is common in a pregnant woman; her muscle tone is reduced, she does less, and because the energy is not burned-up, it is stored as fat deposited in her breasts, on her thighs and on her hips. But the slowing of her body functions has some disadvantages. Her gut is less active, so that her stomach empties more slowly and constipation is common; her kidneys receive a higher concentration of nutrients in her blood stream, and more are filtered out to be lost in the urine. This is part of the price she pays, but it is not difficult for her to compensate for this loss by eating a balanced diet.

The need for the placenta to receive a large quantity of blood, from which to extract the nutrients required by the baby, is met by a 40 per cent increase in the volume of the mother's blood, and by its more rapid circulation through her blood vessels. She manages to achieve this by increasing the amount of blood that the heart pumps out with each beat, and by increasing the rate at which the heart beats. This is why some women are conscious of the action of their heart in pregnancy, and complain of palpitations. More blood is pumped around the body more rapidly. The red blood takes up more oxygen in the lungs, and as nutrients are held longer in the blood stream, these and oxygen can be more readily given to the baby across the placenta.

As has been noted, this exchange takes place through the special cells which form the placenta, and the mother's blood and that of her baby are kept separate at all times. The blood of the fetus passes through its body, then out along the vessels of the umbilical cord and through the network of fine vessels (called capillaries) in the placenta, which you will remember is composed of cells of the outer part of the fertilized egg (see page 120). The tiny vessels are covered by the cells which make up the placenta. Although the placenta resembles a soup-plate when seen after birth, under the microscope it is composed of hundreds of tiny finger-like projections (called villi), each containing the network of tiny capillaries (Fig. **9/12**) through which

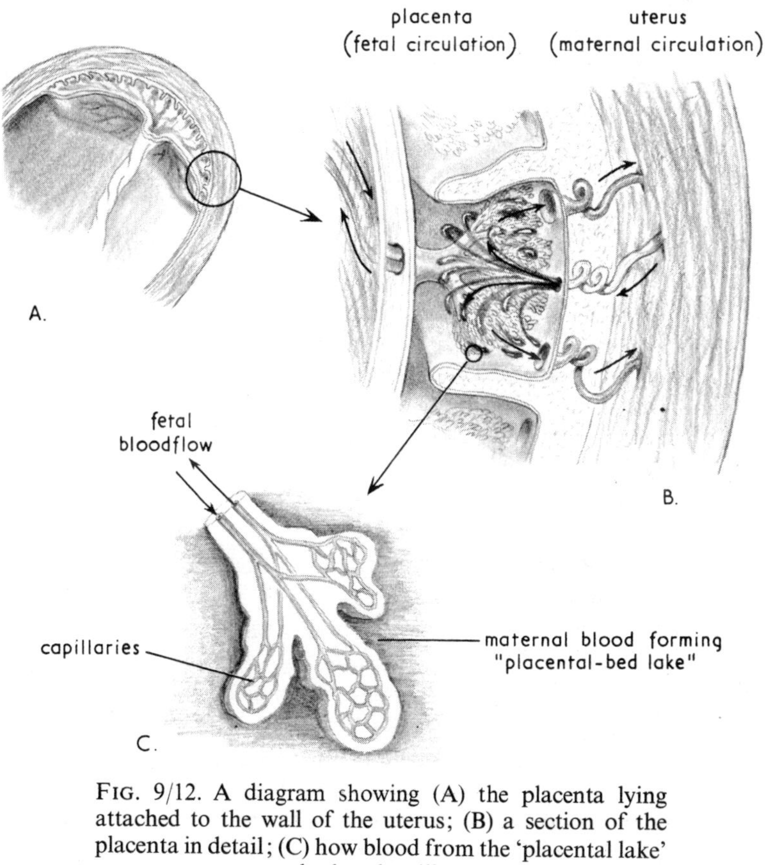

FIG. 9/12. A diagram showing (A) the placenta lying attached to the wall of the uterus; (B) a section of the placenta in detail; (C) how blood from the 'placental lake' bathes the villus

the baby's blood flows. The surface area of these villi is enormous. It has been calculated to be 11 square metres, or 12 square yards. The villi hang into a lake of blood. The lake is filled with blood which comes from the mother's circulation, reaching it by passing through the blood vessels which supply her uterus. The lake lies deep within the uterus, and is in fact lined with tissue made by the placenta, rather as a swimming pool is separated from the garden by a concrete basin. Each time the mother's heart beats, her blood is pumped in spurts into the placental-bed lake, carrying with it the nutrients and oxygen. As it flows between and around the weed-like fronds of the placenta, the oxygen and nutrients are taken from it by the placental cells, and the waste products from the fetus are discharged into the mother's blood stream through the placental cells. In fact, as you can see, the placenta acts as a very efficient lung, kidney and bowel for the fetus.

Cleaned of its waste products and enriched with nutrients and oxygen, the blood in the capillaries of the villi is returned to the fetus along the umbilical vein, and enters its body again at the umbilicus. Meanwhile the mother's blood, with its extra load of waste products, is pumped out of the placental-bed lake and re-enters the mother's circulation to be cleaned by her kidneys, to take up more oxygen from her lungs and nutrients from her gut and liver.

In this way the fetus takes the first pick of what is available to the mother, and even in a famine when the mother is starving, the fetus will get a reasonable amount of food and will not be much underweight at birth.

Other substances also pass across the placenta. For example, if the mother drinks alcohol, some of this crosses the placenta, but does not seem to do the baby any harm. Drugs cross the placenta, so that if the mother is given an antibiotic or an anaesthetic, some of this will appear in the fetus quite quickly. Perhaps more important are the antibodies which cross the placenta. If a person is infected by a germ, he forms substances in his body which attack and destroy the same germ if it infects him again. These substances are called 'antibodies'. Antibodies made by the mother cross the placenta all the time in the second half of pregnancy, so that when the baby is born it has a fair number of antibodies. These protect it against infections which lurk in the environment, until it starts to manufacture its own antibodies, which it does remarkably quickly.

The growth and development of the baby is an astonishing and prodigious event. From a single cell, containing in code all the information needed to make a new individual, growth occurs over a mere 266 days. At the end of this time, a new human being has formed, which is 8 million times heavier than the original fertilized cell. The cells have developed and differentiated to form special tissues and organs, all of which are co-ordinated and working, so that the child can breathe, digest food, move its muscles, hear sounds, taste flavours, react to stimuli, and develop further. A most wondrous growth!

CHAPTER 10

And bears healthy children

It is only in this century that as much attention has been devoted by doctors to the care of the patient during the 40 weeks of pregnancy as was previously paid to the 14 hours of labour. This emphasis on antenatal care has resulted in a very considerable reduction in maternal deaths during childbirth, and a very considerable salvage of babies who might otherwise have died. Good antenatal care is so important that the World Health Organization has had two expert committees consider it. In one report the experts said that the object of antenatal care 'is to ensure that every expectant and nursing mother maintains good health, learns the art of child care, has a normal delivery, and bears healthy children'. In other words, good antenatal care is preventive medicine at its best. But the co-operation of every expectant mother and of her medical adviser is needed to achieve this high standard.

During the antenatal period, the fetus relies upon its mother for all functions, and the healthier the mother, the stronger and healthier will the infant be. Indeed, the health in the first years of life, and maybe even longer, is influenced considerably by the condition of the mother during the prenatal months.

For antenatal care to be effective, the patient must go to her doctor as early as possible in pregnancy, and be seen at regular and increasingly frequent intervals during pregnancy. A good doctor will not only examine the patient, but will provide time so that he may explain the changes occurring in her body, may answer her questions, and banish any anxieties she may have. The patient must always feel that she can ask her doctor about anything that is bothering her. She is not wasting his time, and it is part of the doctor's duty to try and help her, for her emotional condition is as important as her physical condition. Some of the problems about which she may worry are mentioned in this book; but conversation with her doctor is as important as reading, for points which are not properly understood can receive an explanation in conversation.

THE FIRST VISIT

The first visit to the doctor should be made at about the time of the second missed priod. Whether the patient chooses a specialist, or a general practitioner (a personal physician, as he is more properly called) or a doctor in an antenatal clinic, is immaterial. What is important is that she has confidence in her doctor, and that he, for his part, is prepared to seek the opinion of a specialist should this be required. If the patient chooses her personal physician, he will already know a great deal about her general health, and many of the investigations mentioned in this chapter will not be required.

Many women dread the first visit, feeling embarrassed that they will be asked 'personal' questions and examined vaginally. Whilst the questions and examination are necessary, the patient need not be embarrassed, and the doctor will do everything to make the embarrassment as slight as possible. The patient can be reassured that the examination is quite painless.

The questions

The doctor first inquires about the date of the last menstrual period and the duration of the average menstrual cycle. This is measured, as has been mentioned, from the first day of the menstrual period (which is called day 1) to the first day of the next menstrual period. He will also need to know the duration of the menstrual period and whether the character of the bleeding has changed. From this information he can give the patient a prediction of the approximate date of her confinement. The patient can make the calculation herself in this way: to the date of the first day of the last menstrual period add 10 days (counting each month as having 30 days), subtract 3 months from the month in which the period occurred, and add one year. For example, a patient whose menstrual cycle is normal has started her last menstrual period on 12th September, 1970. When will the baby be expected?

Last menstrual period	12 / 9/70
Calculation	+10−3+1
Estimated date of delivery	22 / 6/71

The baby is due on 22nd June, 1971.

Another example: the patient's last menstrual period was 24th April, 1971. When is the baby due? Here the calculation is a bit more complicated, as the addition of 10 days brings the date into another month.

Last menstrual period	24 / 4/71
Add 10 days	+10
	= 4 / 5/71
Subtract 3 months, add 1 year	−3+1
Estimated date of delivery	4 / 2/72

The baby is due on 4th February, 1972.

The estimated date of delivery is accurate to within 14 days in over 80 per cent of women (four woman in every five), and is a great help to the patient in planning for her confinement.

Having told the patient when her baby is expected to be born, the doctor asks how the pregnancy is progressing, and about any complaints the expectant mother may have. He then inquires about her past health, and lists the illnesses and operations which may have occurred. The purpose of these inquiries is to bring to light any conditions which may affect the course of the pregnancy, and for which treatment can be given. If there have been previous pregnancies (including abortions), the doctor should be told about these, and indeed he will inquire searchingly about them in detail. The purpose once again is to try to anticipate complications, and to find out how well (or badly) the patient was able to cope with her previous pregnancies.

The examination

The remainder of the visit is taken up with the examination. For this it is usual for the patient to strip completely and to put on a gown provided by the doctor. This is important, as the doctor tries to find out the general health of the patient. Usually he first notes her height and records her weight. Then he examines her breasts, and determines if the nipples are normal. If she proposes to breast-feed her baby, he may prescribe certain manipulations which are done by the patient herself during pregnancy. These manipulations encourage milk production and make the establishment of breast-feeding easier. He then listens to the patient's heart with a stethoscope, gently palpates her abdomen, and observes her legs to see if there are any varicose veins. In early pregnancy, the abdominal palpation is merely to check the tone of the abdominal muscles and to see whether there is any enlargement of the liver or spleen. After the 12th week of pregnancy, the doctor also palpates the enlarging uterus to determine if the baby is growing normally, and after the 28th week to check the position of the baby in the womb. After these examinations, and prior to the pelvic examination, the doctor takes the patient's blood pressure. It is left until this stage as emotions can often cause a rise in the blood pressure, and the doctor is trying to obtain a baseline blood pressure against which to measure changes. The estimation of the blood pressure is a most important investigation and is made at every visit, since a rise in blood pressure in pregnancy warns the doctor that 'toxaemia of pregancy' may be starting. Its exact cause is not known, but it is known that the arteries which supply the uterus and the kidneys go into a spasm. If the spasm becomes severe, the blood supply to the placenta is reduced, and the baby may fail to grow properly, or may even die in the womb. The severity of the spasm can be reduced if 'toxaemia of pregnancy' is detected early. Appropriate treatment at this time will control the disease before it becomes a danger to the well-being of the baby.

Finally, the doctor performs a pelvic examination. It was noted in Chapter 8 that this examination is neither painful nor embarrassing if the patient co-operates. The doctor first introduces a speculum into the vagina to inspect the cervix and to take the 'Pap smear'. He then gently performs a pelvic examination with two fingers introduced into the vagina.

Laboratory investigations

No first antenatal visit can be considered complete until the doctor has made certain laboratory tests. Just before the pelvic examination, the doctor will have asked his patient to empty her bladder of urine. Many doctors ask for the urine to be passed in a special way. The patient is given a small moist cotton-wool swab with which she cleans the entrance to her vagina, wiping from the front backwards. She then starts to urinate, and when the flow of urine is running, she collects the 'midstream' specimen in a sterile container which has been given to her. This method is only necessary at the first visit. At all other visits, the patient either brings the urine specimen with her, or passes it into a container in the normal way. The purpose of the midstream specimen is to enable the doctor to find out if the patient has a hidden infection of the urinary tract. This hidden infection often becomes obvious in pregnancy, causing kidney infection, and many doctors believe in giving prophylactic treatment. The specimen of urine is also examined for the presence of protein and sugar. The presence of the former is another sign of impending 'toxaemia of pregnancy'. If sugar is found in the urine, investigations are made to find out if the patient has sugar diabetes.

Several important tests are made on a sample of blood taken from a vein in the arm. Patients tend to fear this procedure, but the discomfort is only momentary and the information obtained is very valuable. The blood is examined by a special test to determine if the patient has syphilis. This disease, which is spread by coitus, is increasing in incidence. It is important to detect the disease early in pregnancy when its cure is relatively easy. If left untreated, syphilis can damage the baby severely. In late pregnancy, the germs which cause syphilis pass through the placenta and multiply in the fetal tissues, either killing the fetus or damaging some of its organs. Those children who are the victims of congenital syphilis can be treated after birth, but treatment is not always successful. But if the disease is detected in early pregnancy and treated adequately, congenital syphilis will be prevented.

The specimen of blood is also examined to find out the mother's blood group, particularly whether she is Rhesus negative. Rhesus disease is considered in Chapter 16.

Finally, a sample of the blood taken, or else a further finger-prick specimen of blood, is examined to estimate the haemoglobin concentration. The haemoglobin concentration measures the amount of iron in the red blood cells, and so is an index of anaemia. It is important for the doctor to know if anaemia is present, as the expectant mother requires extra iron because the fetus also has to obtain a considerable amount of iron from the mother during pregnancy. If the haemoglobin concentration is low, the doctor will be able to treat it before it has any serious effects. Since the baby takes most of its iron requirements in late pregnancy, the haemoglobin estimation is repeated twice more during pregnancy, at the 32nd week, when the baby is beginning to increase its demand for iron, and again at the 36th week. Thus if the mother has become anaemic, she can be treated adequately before her confinement.

The summing-up

The examination and tests are over, the expectant mother has dressed again, has made-up her face, and now sits talking to her doctor so that he can discuss the diet she should eat, the exercise she should take, and can clear up any doubts she may have. She should not hesitate to ask her doctor about any matter which is bothering her. All too often, alas, women obtain misinformation about pregnancy from acquaintances, whose experiences invariably seem to have been gruesome. Just as after surgical operations, many women revel in exaggerating their experiences or, what is worse, misinterpreting the experiences they think that their friends have had. These women are all too ready to offer gratuitous information and advice to expectant mothers. Much of the information is erroneous, much of the advice harmful, so that the expectant mother is anxious, bewildered and confused. The person to clear up her confusion is the doctor. She should ignore the gossip of well-meaning busybodies, and should feel able to ask her doctor for accurate information at all times. He, for his part, should always be ready, and have time, to discuss the pregnancy with the expectant mother.

SUBSEQUENT VISITS

If she is otherwise normal, the expectant mother will make an antenatal visit to her doctor every 4 weeks until she is 28 weeks pregnant (7 lunar months), every 2 weeks from then until she is 36 weeks pregnant (9 lunar months), and every week from then until she has been confined. If any complication arises, or if the patient has previously had some illness, such as diabetes, 'blood pressure' or a heart condition, the doctor will want to see her more frequently.

At each of the visits during pregnancy, the doctor is concerned about two people–the expectant mother who is carrying the baby, and the fetus as it floats weightless in its heat-controlled, waste-disposal and food-intake controlled capsule (the amniotic sac) within the uterus. At each visit the doctor will seek to find out how the patient is progressing, and how she is enjoying her pregnancy. He will answer any queries, and if he detects that all is not progressing normally, will give advice. At each visit the expectant mother's weight is noted, and a weight gain of more than 4.5 kg. (9 lb.) in the first 20 weeks, or more than 0·5 kg. (1 lb.) a week in each of the last 20 weeks is usually frowned upon. Some doctors get most upset if the weight gain between visits exceeds these figures. The ankles and legs are examined for swelling and varicose veins, the blood pressure is recorded, and the urine tested.

The doctor then turns his attention to the baby. He estimates the height of the uterus, as was described previously, and he palpates it gently to find out the exact position of the baby. He will probably find that up to the 28th week (7th lunar month), the baby will be in a different position each time. It may be head down (called a cephalic presentation), or with its head in the upper part of the uterus and the buttocks in the lower part (a breech presentation), or it may be cross-ways (a transverse or shoulder presentation) (Fig. **10/1**). This is because at this early stage of pregnancy there is a relatively large volume of 'water' (really amniotic fluid, which does not have quite the same composition as water) in the amniotic sac, and the baby can therefore move about easily. After the 30th week of pregnancy, the great majority of babies settle with their head over the mother's pelvis, and their buttocks in the wider upper part of the uterus. By the 40th week–also called 'term'–96 per cent of babies lie in this position, as cephalic presentations, and between 3 and 4 per cent lie as breech presentations. In some cases the back of the baby is on the right side of the uterus, and in others on the left. It makes little difference to the progress of labour, and the baby can change positions between two examinations. The gentle palpation of the uterus distinguishes these points, and enables the doctor to determine whether the baby is lying as a cephalic or a breech presentation (Fig. **10/2**). This is of some importance at about the 34th week, as

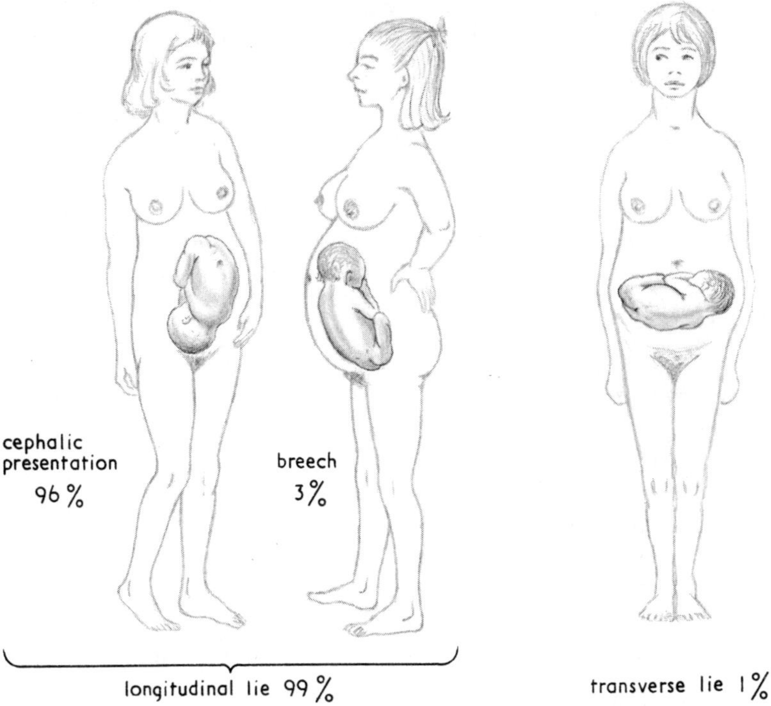

FIG. 10/1. How the baby lies in the uterus. The percentages given for the different presentations are those found just before labour begins

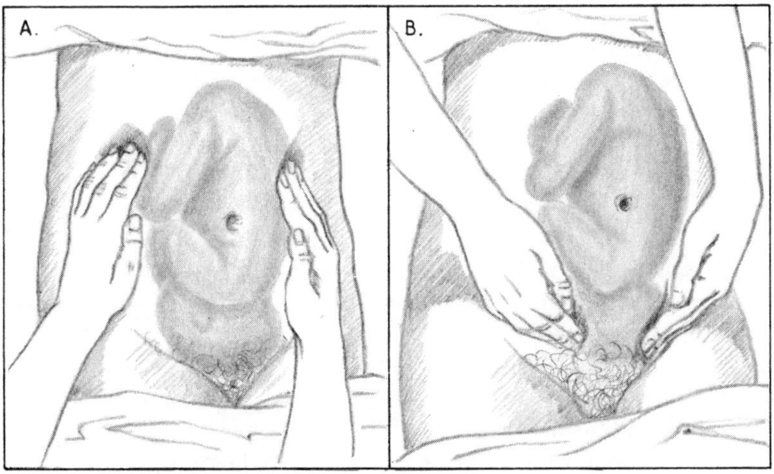

FIG. 10/2. How the doctor finds the position of the baby. (A) Feeling the back; (B) Detecting the baby's head

the doctor may wish to try to 'turn' the breech baby into a cephalic presentation with head down. At every visit the doctor should tell the expectant mother where the baby is, and should help her to feel it if she wishes. If he listens to the baby's heart, and she wishes to hear her baby's heart beat, he should try to arrange for her to do this using his stethoscope. The baby's heart beats much faster than the mother's, averaging 120 beats a minute, but varying a bit.

Lightening

By the end of the 36th week, most women carrying their first baby (primigravidae) feel 'lightening'. This is because the baby's head 'drops' into the pelvic cavity; consequently the upper part of the uterus drops, relieving the pressure under the ribs and making breathing easier. Lightening often occurs suddenly, the expectant mother waking up one morning relieved of the pressure and discomfort she has experienced previously. Unfortunately, the descent of the head into the pelvic cavity is often associated with pressure on the pelvis, and an increased vaginal discharge, so that she exchanges one set of mild complaints for another. At this time, too, the painless uterine contractions which have been felt for some weeks become more frequent.

In women who have had previous children, 'lightening' takes place later, either in the week or 10 days before labour starts or in the early stages of labour.

Pelvic examination

The descent of the fetal head into the pelvic cavity is a good indication that the pelvic size and shape are normal. The doctor uses this information to be sure that this is so. It is usual for him to make a pelvic examination at the 37th week. At this examination, he assesses the size of the pelvis, the relationship of the fetal head to the pelvic brim, and the softness and degree of opening of the cervix. The examination is delayed until this stage of pregnancy for two reasons: firstly, the fetal head has usually descended into the pelvis (doctors call this 'engagement' of the fetal head); and secondly, the pelvic tissues at this time are soft and stretch easily, so that the examination is painless. Just as she did during the pelvic examination at the first antenatal visit, the patient must relax her muscles completely in order for the doctor to obtain the maximum information.

The last weeks of pregnancy

The antenatal visits are made at weekly intervals; the patient has learned what signs show that labour has started; she is confident about her doctor; she is fit and well; she has a knowledge of what happens in labour; she has prepared the baby's clothes; she has visited the hospital; and the doctor has answered all her questions. In short, she is a healthy, knowledgeable mother, who has learned the art of child care, who knows the sequence of events she may expect in labour, and she is about to have a normal delivery and bear a healthy child.

CHAPTER 11

An ABC of hygiene in pregnancy

The conditions discussed in this chapter are all 'minor', that is they are minor in that they do not cause serious disease. To the expectant mother they may be major problems. Since so many body systems may be involved, it seems appropriate to list the conditions alphabetically for more ready reference.

ALCOHOL

There is no reason why the expectant mother should not drink alcohol in moderate amounts if she so wishes. It has not been found to affect the course of pregnancy adversely, and indeed there is some evidence that alcohol prevents premature labour. However, this is not a reason for recommending alcohol for other than moderate social drinking.

BACKACHE

In late pregnancy particularly, the pelvic joints and ligaments relax. At the same time the growing weight of the uterus changes the centre of balance, so that the expectant mother has to stand with her shoulders further back than normal. This position has been called 'the pride of pregnancy'. However, it and the relaxed ligaments produce backache to some extent in most pregnant women, but more so in multigravidae (pregnant women who have previously had one or more pregnancies). The backache increases during the day and is felt most towards evening, and at night when it may prevent sleep. The pain is usually felt low in the back or over the sacro-iliac joint. Treatment is largely to prevent the condition from becoming severe. If the expectant mother's posture is bad, she should seek advice.

High heels tend to aggravate the strain on the back, and should be avoided except when going out. 'Flatties' are fine in the house. If the backache is marked, analgesics may be needed, but the doctor should be consulted first.

BATHING

Showers are recommended in preference to long baths (or tub baths, as the Americans call them) in the last four weeks of pregnancy, when the bath water may conceivably enter the vagina. Before this time long baths are perfectly safe and pleasantly relaxing! Swimming in general is permissible, and may be continued as near term as the expectant mother wishes.

BREASTS

Care of the breasts in pregnancy helps the establishment of breast-feeding. The nipples should be stroked and drawn out gently for about two minutes a day from early pregnancy. If the expectant mother wishes, she may rub in some bland lanolin ointment, particularly if the nipples are dry. From about the 32nd week (8th lunar month), the breasts should be 'expressed' by placing both hands with the palms widely spread around them, and pressing towards the nipples. It will be found that a yellow secretion appears. This manipulation is thought to keep the ducts of the breasts open (Fig. **11/1**).

CLOTHING

What should a pregnant woman wear? She should wear the clothes in which she is her most attractive, but which are comfortable at the same time. She will need a larger sized, well-fitting brassière because of the enlargement of her breasts due to pregnancy, and may wish to wear a maternity girdle, but expensive, complicated pregnancy 'foundation' garments are quite unnecessary. An ordinary elastic maternity girdle is all that is needed, and even this is not essential if the expectant mother feels comfortable without one. She should avoid constricting garters or elastic-topped stockings, as these may interfere with the return of blood from the legs in pregnancy, so

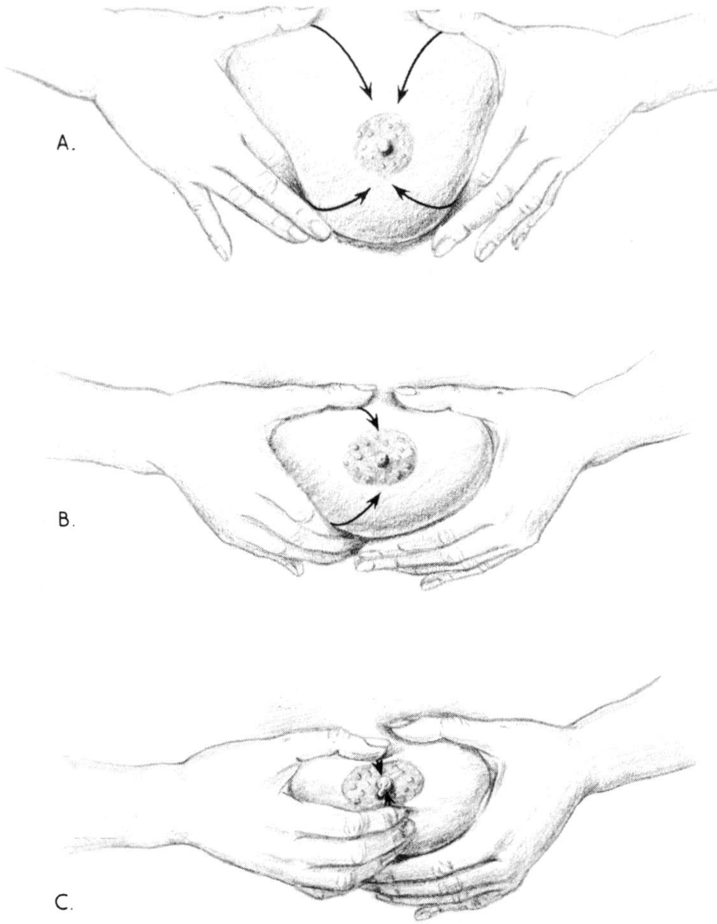

FIG. 11/1. The care of the breasts in pregnancy
A. How the hands are placed at the start of expression, to enclose the breast at its margin
B. The hands move inwards towards the areola, firm pressure is exerted on the whole breast. The movement is repeated about 5 to 10 times
C. The breast is fixed by one hand and the milk ducts are compressed with the other hand, the thumb above and the fingers below. The pressure empties the milk ducts. At the end of the expression, the nipple is drawn out with the fingers

increasing the risk of varicose veins, but a panty-girdle or pantyhose is quite suitable. When at home or working, she should wear low-heeled shoes, but if she goes out to some special event, she can wear normal high-heeled shoes. The pregnant woman should aim to look as attractive as possible, and not be a frump!

COITUS

If the expectant mother's pregnancy is normal and she has no tendency to premature labour or repeated abortions, sexual intercourse may continue at a frequency which is normal for that couple. Some women find that they desire more frequent coitus in pregnancy; others find they are less stimulated. Coitus should be gentle, at all times, and in the second half of pregnancy the wife may find that penile entry from the rear, the wife lying in front of her husband, is more comfortable and satisfying.

CONSTIPATION

You have two kinds of muscle in your body – the voluntary striped muscles, and the involuntary smooth muscles. The striped muscles make up the muscles of your arms and legs, and respond to your control. If you want to pick up a saucepan, a message goes from your brain and your arm muscles move your hand forward. If you find the saucepan is too hot, you voluntarily stop the movement! The smooth muscles make up the muscles of your heart, your gut, and your womb. These muscles work without voluntary control, and you cannot voluntarily alter their action. However, they do respond to some drugs and hormones. Progesterone, the special hormone of pregnancy, relaxes smooth muscle. In one way this is useful, as it enables the uterus (which is mainly composed of smooth muscle) to grow without attempting to expel the fetus prematurely. In other ways smooth muscle relaxation can be annoying. The muscle tone of the gut is lowered throughout pregnancy, which leads to constipation. In late pregnancy, the tendency is aggravated by pressure on the lower bowel by the enlarged uterus. If the expectant mother is worried about constipation, she should increase her fluid intake, and re-establish the 'habit' by attempting to open her bowels regularly just after a meal. If these methods fail, her doctor will give her

'Senokot' (Standardised Senna) or the contact stool-softening laxative, bisacodyl. She should avoid self-medication with strong laxatives, or oily laxatives.

DENTAL CARE

Care of the teeth does not differ in pregnancy from that at other times. The old notion that each child cost a tooth is a relic from the time when regular visits to the dentist were not made. Unfortunately, particularly in Australia, this still applies. In areas where fluoride is not added to the drinking-water, the use of one tablet per day containing 1 mg. fluorine taken from the 20th week of pregnancy will protect the infant against dental caries. A few women develop swelling of the gums at the base of the teeth (marginal gingivitis, as it is called). This is not abnormal, and disappears after childbirth, but if in any doubt the expectant mother should consult a dentist.

DIET

More rubbish has been written about diet in pregnancy than on almost any other medical subject. In the years before World War II, the influence of diet on the growth and survival of the baby was thought to be considerable. Recent studies have cast doubt on this, and present opinion is that within the normal range of diets available, their influence on the birth weight and survival of the baby is minimal. As far as the obstetrical efficiency of the expectant mother is concerned, the diet she ate in her own infancy and childhood has much more importance. This is the reason the World Health Organization's Expert Committee on Maternity Care said that one of the objectives of antenatal care was to help the expectant mother 'learn the art of child care'. This includes giving her child a properly balanced diet, rich in protein.

By and large then, the effect of diet on the outcome of pregnancy has been exaggerated in the past. Fanciful, vague, complicated diets have been ordered which had little value and were often confusing. I do not suggest that a pregnant woman should not pay attention to what she eats. She should! In pregnancy she has to provide the nutrients necessary for the growth of her child, as well as for her own needs. This does not mean that she needs to 'eat for two', and as will be seen later, *excessive weight gained in pregnancy is very hard to take off*. It does mean that she should understand what she is eating and why.

Basically the diet provides *carbohydrates and fat*, which produce the energy needed for life; *protein*, needed for the formation of new tissues; *vitamins and minerals*, which help in the complex chemical processes in the body. All foodstuffs contain one or more of the above nutrients. Unfortunately, the cheaper foodstuffs are the energy-supplying carbohydrates, whilst the tissue-building protein, the vitamins and some of the minerals come from relatively expensive foods, like meat. Because of this, poorer people, and most of the people in the developing countries, eat too little protein, vitamins and minerals, and barely enough carbohydrate to provide the energy needed for their daily tasks. This energy is measured in a unit called a calorie, and the average pregnant woman needs about 2,500 calories a day. In the affluent lands, most women eat too much, particularly carbohydrates such as bread, cakes, sweets and sugar, but often eat only just enough protein. Their calorie intake is excessive for their needs, and the excess is stored in the body as fat.

Pregnancy puts an increased demand for protein, and unless the expectant mother alters to a diet which provides more protein, she may not get sufficient, whilst still eating too much carbohydrate.

The nutritional needs of a pregnant woman have been considered in great detail by high-powered committees in many countries, and the optimal, or best, daily allowance for a woman weighing about 55 kg. (121 lb.) has been worked out to be:

Calories	2500
Protein	65 g.
Calcium	1000 mg.
Iron	15 mg.
Vitamin A	6000 u.
Vitamin D	400 u.
Vitamin B:	
Thiamine	1·0 mg.
Riboflavine	1·5 mg.
Nicotinic Acid	15·0 mg.
Vitamin C (Ascorbic acid)	50·0 mg.
Folic acid	0·3 mg.

To the average expectant mother, the above table is so much

jargon, but it can easily be translated into foodstuffs. This is shown in Table **11/1**, and is summarized here: (1) *Dairy products:* The expectant mother should drink 1 to 1½ pints of milk a day, either raw or made up in drinks or used in cooking. If she wants, she can substitue cheese for milk, 1 ounce being equivalent to ½ pint. (2) *Meat and eggs:* She should eat 2 to 4 ounces of meat, fish or poultry a day, and usually have an egg. (3) *Vegetables:* She should eat green leafy vegetables, cooked for less than 10 minutes in a minimum of water, at least three times a week, and other vegetables as she wishes. (4) *Bread, cereals, sugar, sweets, potatoes:* These provide the energy, but in excess these are the ones which put on the weight. Some carbohydrate is needed, but as the expectant mother has to pay attention to her weight, she should eat these sparingly. (5) *Fruits:* She should eat an orange or a grapefruit each day, and any additional fresh fruit she fancies.

Table 11/1

Nutritional Needs in Pregnancy

Food		*Calories*	*Protein (g.)*
Dairy products	A daily total of 600–900 ml. (1 to 1½ pints) of milk, either raw or used in cooking or in hot drinks. Cheese can be substituted, 30 g. (1 oz.) being equal to 300 ml. (½ pint) of milk.	600	32
	Butter or margarine can be taken as required (say 60 g., or 2 oz.).	480	—
Meat Products	The meat product may be *lean* meat, poultry, fish or liver. A serving of 60–120 g. (2–4 oz.) a day will provide for the needs. More meat may, of course, be eaten if desired. It is best grilled, roasted or stewed, rather than fried.	250	20

Food		*Calories*	*Protein (g.)*
Egg	One a day (or at least most days).	90	6
Bread and other cereals (including sugar as required)	Three to four slices, which is equal to 120 g. (4 oz.) is probably sufficient. A half-full teacup of breakfast cereal equals one slice of bread. Wholemeal bread is preferable to white flour bread.	320	10
	Sugar or jam, say 60 g. or 2 oz.	240	—
Vegetables	*Potato:* One to two medium-sized potatoes (150–300 g., or 5–10 oz.). The potato can be cooked in any way, but the most nutritious are those cooked in their skin. If desired, potatoes can be replaced by squash, pumpkin or turnips. In working out a diet, the bread and potato are interchangeable.	140	5
	Vegetables: Salads and other green or yellow leafy vegetables, peas, beans and lentils contain valuable vitamins if they are cooked properly. About 60–120 g. (2–4 oz.) should be eaten daily.	50	3
Fruit	The old adage 'an apple a day keeps the doctor away' applies in pregnancy. For variety, the apple can be replaced by citrus fruits (orange, grapefruit) or by tomato juice, which are all rich in Vitamin C.	50	1
		2260	77

How she divides up the foodstuffs, having what at which meal, must be her decision. How well, or badly, she cooks the food is the result of her upbringing. How efficiently she chooses and buys the proper foods is the result of her education. If a mother wishes her child to be a good housekeeper, she will have the opportunity over the years to teach her, and this teaching will be reinforced in the schools. To start the lessons, the expectant mother can remember most of what is needed about diet and nutrition in pregnancy if she recalls the following slogan: 'Buy all you can afford from the butcher, the greengrocer and at the dairy; spend only little at the confectioner, the grocer and the chemist'.

DOUCHING

Vaginal douching is a peculiarly American habit, founded on an exaggerated need for so-called 'personal hygiene'. The vagina is self-cleansing. Douches are usually unnecessary at any time, and particularly in pregnancy, when they have a slight danger. So do not douche!

DRUGS IN PREGNANCY

After the 'thalidomide' tragedy, doctors have been even more careful in prescribing drugs to pregnant women. It will be remembered that thalidomide was given in early pregnancy as a sedative or to alleviate nausea. Later it was found that it had prevented the development of the arm and leg buds of the fetus, so that the affected babies were born alive but without arms or legs.

No new drugs are now prescribed for pregnant women unless they have been investigated by the most exhaustive tests, and most doctors only give expectant mothers drugs which they *really* need. The mother herself, particularly in the first 12 weeks of pregnancy, should avoid taking any drug unless she has checked with her doctor, and then only if it is really required.

Today, the expectant mother can rest assured that none of the drugs commonly prescribed during pregnancy has any damaging action on her growing baby.

EMPLOYMENT

Provided that the expectant mother enjoys her work and that it does not subject her to too great a physical strain, the job may be continued throughout pregnancy. In many countries legislation has been enacted which gives paid maternity leave for the last 6 to 8 weeks of pregnancy. After delivery it is usual to be given paid leave from work for 4 to 6 weeks, so that the baby may be cared for, and the mother may adjust to her new duties.

EXERCISE

Pregnancy is a normal event and should be treated as such. Exercise should be encouraged if this is the usual habit of the patient, but if the expectant mother normally takes no exercise beyond housework, she need not change her habits. The average woman takes a reasonable amount of exercise, and can continue to take it in pregnancy. If she enjoys swimming, she may swim. If she plays tennis or golf, she may continue until the enlarging uterus prevents accurately placed strokes! If she enjoys walking or gardening, then she should continue to walk or garden. In general, she need not alter the pattern of exercise to which she is accustomed, just because she is pregnant.

FAINTING

Fainting attacks, palpitations and headaches occasionally occur in pregnancy, and are due to the alterations in the expectant mother's circulatory system produced by the pregnancy. Although annoying, they have no sinister significance, and in Victorian days a faint was the way the modest wife announced to her husband that 'a little stranger was on the way'!

FREQUENCY OF URINATION

Irritability of the bladder is quite common in early pregnancy, and once again in the last weeks when the baby's head presses into the pelvis. Nothing much can be done about it, except to pass urine more often. If urination is associated with pain and scalding, the expectant mother should consult her doctor.

HAEMORRHOIDS

Haemorrhoids, or piles, are not infrequently found in pregnancy. They are more common in multigravidae, and seem to occur in families. The usual complaints are of bleeding during a bowel motion, the presence of a tender lump noticed during the use of toilet paper, or pain. Constipation and straining to empty the bowels aggravate these complaints. The expectant mother can reduce the discomfort of haemorrhoids by avoiding constipation, and making sure that the stool is never hard. Her doctor will be able to prescribe ointments which relieve the pain and reduce the swelling of prolapsed piles.

HEARTBURN

Heartburn is an annoying and fairly common complaint, which is more frequent in late pregnancy. It is due to the passage of small amounts of stomach contents into the lower part of the food tube (or oesophagus), which leads from the mouth to the stomach. In pregnancy this occurs because the valve guarding the entrance to the stomach relaxes, and because the enlarging uterus pushes up against the stomach. It is often worse at night, when the burning sensation in the upper abdomen can be quite distressing. Despite its name, it can be seen that heartburn has nothing to do with the heart. The expectant mother can relieve heartburn by eating small meals more frequently, and by taking a glass of milk to bed with her, and sipping this if heartburn occurs. She would also be wise to sleep propped up on one or two extra pillows. If heartburn persists, her doctor will prescribe one of the many antacid tablets or liquids. The more modern ones, based on aluminium or magnesium, are preferable to those containing sodium (salt), such as sodium bicarbonate, as this increases the patient's intake of salt, which may not be advisable.

IMMUNIZATION

Apart from immunization or vaccination against smallpox, which should be avoided in the first half of pregnancy, immunization programmes can be carried out as required. Indeed, because of the apparently increased risk of poliomyelitis to pregnant women, the expectant mother should be immunized against this disease if she has not previously taken her Sabin vaccine. Since the vaccine is given by mouth, it is quite painless and devoid of side-effects. There is a belief, too, that pregnant women are more susceptible to chest complications of influenza, and many doctors recommend that pregnant women should receive anti-influenza injections if an epidemic is expected. I am doubtful of the truth of this, as so many strains of the influenza virus exist, that the injection may only protect the patient (if it does) against one. Moreover, the injections are painful. In case of doubt, the patient should consult her own doctor. It is possible that a safe, painless, effective anti-influenzal vaccine may be developed soon which can be sprayed into the nose. If this happens, the views I have expressed can be ignored.

LEG CRAMPS

Some expectant mothers develop leg cramps in late pregnancy. These occur mostly at night, and the cause is not known. Treatment is not very satisfactory, and there is some evidence that excessive milk intake may be the cause. This is why the total milk intake recommended was 1 to 1½ pints. If the patient has leg cramps, a drink of milk from the allowance may help. However, the evidence that excessive milk is the cause of leg cramps is not very secure, as leg cramps occur in Asian women who do not habitually drink milk.

MATERNAL PRENATAL INFLUENCES

A considerable literature has grown up about how maternal influences can affect the baby. This obstetric superstition has been propagated from antiquity, and sought to explain the birth of deformed or blemished infants. This tribal myth has been used by playwrights and novelists to tell dramatic stories, and is still widely believed. It has, of course, no substance. There is no evidence that maternal impressions can in any way affect the baby. The reasons are many: firstly, there is no nervous connection between the mother and her baby; secondly, the blood of the mother is quite separate from that of the baby; and thirdly, the infant is completely formed by the 8th week of pregnancy, so that for the impression to have any effect it must occur before this time. In most cases, the 'shocking experience' which the mother 'knows' is the cause of her baby's birth defect occurred much later. The truth is that maternal impressions have no effect on the growth or development of the baby. The baby will not become a famous television actor if the expectant mother spends hours watching television. The infant will not be exceptionally gifted musically if the mother persistently listens to, or plays, music during pregnancy; nor will he be a famous sportsman if her husband insists that she watches all the ball games she can over the 40 weeks of pregnancy; nor will the sight of a one-eyed black cat crossing the road mean that her baby will be born one-eyed and black!

It is true that a few babies are born with congenital defects, but the number with a defect is less than three in every hundred. This means that 97 of every 100 babies born are perfectly formed, and of the three which have defects, most can be treated. But it is not true that the defects are due to prenatal influences. They are usually due to an inherited defect in one of the genes which make up the new individual. Occassionally, however, they are due to infection by the rubella virus occurring during pregnancy. This is the virus which causes German measles, and the problem is discussed further on page 223.

NAUSEA

About 50 per cent of pregnant women experience some degree of nausea, and a few vomit. This complaint occurs in the first 12 weeks of pregnancy, disappearing at the end of this time, but sometimes recurring in late pregnancy. The cause is almost certainly a sensitivity to the hormones of pregnancy, but the condition may be exaggerated if the expectant mother is over-anxious or emotionally stressed. Most often the nausea occurs in the morning, hence the name 'morning sickness', but it may occur at any time of the day. Nausea in the morning is more common than at other times of the day, because the stomach contains the overnight accumulation of gastric juices.

Most women are able to overcome the nausea by simple means. The constitution of the diet should be adjusted to exclude greasy, fatty foods, and fried foods should be avoided. Small carbohydrate-rich meals are taken at more frequent intervals, the first being brought to the wife by her husband as soon as possible after waking. This may consist of toast or biscuits, and tea. After this, small meals are eaten every 3 hours until bedtime. Some women find it better to avoid drinking at meals and to take the fluids, either as sweetened fruit drinks, weak tea or milk and soda-water, at other times.

An example of a suitable diet for the day is:

On waking	A slice of toast or two Cream Cracker biscuits, with a drink of weak tea.
8.00 a.m.	Light breakfast of cereal, or toast with honey or jam, and perhaps weak tea. If the expectant mother feels she can eat more, she adjusts the diet to her own needs.
10.00 a.m.	Toast with a glass of milk, tea or a fruit drink.
12.30 p.m.	Lunch. Soup with toast or Cream Crackers; rice or noodles with lightly boiled vegetables.
3.30 p.m.	Tea. Toast, jam, fruit juice, and perhaps plain cake.
6.30 p.m.	Dinner. Lean meat or chicken, green vegetables, potatoes, salad and rice pudding.
9.30 p.m.	A drink of tea, cocoa, warm milk, or milk and soda.
To bed	A drink and Cream Crackers to take if the expectant mother wakes up during the night.

This is only an example, and a great number of variations can be chosen by the individual herself. If the nausea is troublesome, the expectant mother should consult her doctor. Although many and varied drugs have been prescribed in the past, doctors today are very wary of new drugs in early pregnancy. However, two kinds of drugs are safe and fairly effective; one is a barbiturate derivative, and the other an antihistamine.

NOSE BLEEDS

Slight bleeding from the nose is not unusual in pregnancy. It is due to the increased blood supply which occurs, and in most cases needs no treatment. It does not mean that the expectant mother has a high blood pressure.

PICA

For some reason, which the psychiatrists try to explain, bizarre cravings for strange foods may occur in pregnancy. Unfortunately, each group of psychiatrists has a different explanation, so the *fact* of bizarre cravings remains, but the *reason* remains unknown. If the craving is for substances other than foodstuffs, the craving is called 'pica'. The word comes from the Latin term for 'magpie', a bird which collects strange articles. Severe craving is not very common, and true pica is rather rare. Most women who do have cravings want carbohydrates (either sweets or laundry starch), or large amounts of fruit. A few have cravings for more exotic things, such as pickles, caviare or avocados. The very few who have true pica may urgently crave to eat coal, clay or pencils. If the expectant mother develops strange cravings for foods in pregnancy, she must realize that she is not going mad, but that the cravings exist and need to be controlled.

PLACIDITY

To the annoyance of the intellectually alert expectant mother, she notes an increasing placidity and drowsiness as pregnancy advances. She no longer has the clarity of mind and precision of thought she had before pregnancy. Even small intellectual matters become a trial; to do anything is an effort and she fears she is becoming bovine. The cause is the increased circulation of the pregnancy hormone progesterone. and she can be reassured that the placidity will pass once the baby is born. Meanwhile. she will have to look inwards into the warmth of her womb, rather than attempting to equal Einstein!

SHORTNESS OF BREATH

In late pregnancy a number of expectant mothers find that even moderate exertion causes shortness of breath. Provided their doctor has checked that their heart and lungs are normal, the shortness of breath, although inconvenient, is without danger.

SMOKING

The influence of cigarette smoking on pregnancy has been studied in the last few years. The evidence at present is that cigarette smoking, particularly if more than 10 cigarettes are smoked per day, has an adverse effect on pregnancy. There seems to be an increased risk that abortion will occur, and the birth weight of the baby is likely to be less than that of a baby born to a woman who does not smoke. Expectant mothers should avoid excessive smoking during pregnancy, although as far as the baby is concerned, less than 10 cigarettes a day can be smoked without any harm. However, smoking is a probable cause of lung cancer, and pregnancy might be a good time to stop smoking altogether.

SWEATING

In late pregnancy, many expectant mothers find that they sweat more easily and in hot, humid weather 'feel the heat intolerably'. Sometimes night sweats occur, the expectant mother waking up in a 'lather of sweat'. The excessive sweating is due to dilated blood vessels in the skin, which in turn dilate because of pregnancy. No specific treatment is available, and all that the expectant mother can do is to avoid excessive exertion, to take frequent rest periods, and have frequent cool showers. Because if the increased fluid lost by sweating, the expectant mother should increase her fluid intake.

SWELLING OF THE ANKLES AND LEGS (OEDEMA)

Retention of fluid in the tissues of the body is normal in pregnancy. The average expectant mother retains between 3 and 6 litres ($6\frac{1}{2}$ to 13 pints) of fluid, half of it in the last 10 weeks of pregnancy. Swelling of the ankles, the lowest part of the body, is therefore common. If it occurs in the evening, it is not serious, and all that the expectant mother needs to do is keep her feet up. Women who are overweight for their height by the 20th week of pregnancy, and overweight women who gain more than 0.5 kg. (1.1 lb.) per week after the 30th week, have almost a 50 per cent chance of developing evening oedema. In general this is unimportant, but if these women, and all others, develop swelling of the legs earlier in the day, it is a warning sign that 'toxaemia of pregnancy' may be developing, and the mother-to-be should hasten to see her doctor.

TRAVEL

Apart from the restriction by airlines on carrying women more than 32 weeks pregnant who have no certificate of fitness from their doctor, an expectant mother can travel wherever she likes during pregnancy. She may safely travel by aeroplane, by ship or by car – or at least as safely as other motorists will let her! The only problem may be that she may go into labour at her destination, and will have to find a new obstetrician.

URINARY TRACT INFECTION

About 5 per cent of women have a hidden infection of the urinary tract, which causes them no trouble until they become pregnant. In pregnancy, owing to the muscle-relaxing effects of progesterone, the collecting area in the kidney and the tube which connects the kidney to the bladder become larger. Urine tends to stagnate in these areas, and in the bladder. Women who have hidden urinary tract infection (called 'bacteriuria'), unless treated, have twice the chance of developing anaemia, a raised blood pressure, and of delivering a 'premature baby'. It is usual for doctors to examine the urine in early pregnancy for the presence of bacteriuria, and if this is found, to give treatment. This treatment will also prevent the onset of kidney infection, or pyelonephritis. The collecting area of the kidney is called the renal pelvis, or *pyelos* (a Greek word meaning a trough). If the urine becomes infected, the kidney pyelos and the kidney tissue itself may become inflamed – which is why this type of kidney infection is called pyelonephritis.

The symptoms of pyelonephritis are pain in the loins, fever and shivering, sweating, and painful urination. Should these symptoms occur in pregnancy, the expectant mother should call her doctor without delay, as treatment using sulfa drugs or antibiotics is very successful.

VAGINAL DISCHARGE

During pregnancy the normal secretions which keep the vagina moist are increased, and additional secretions derived from the glands of the cervix add to the quantity. About 30 per cent of expectant mothers are conscious of the increased vaginal discharge. If the quantity necessitates the wearing of a pad, the mother-to-be should consult her doctor, so that investigations may be undertaken to determine if the discharge is merely an exaggeration of the normal; if it is due to infection by the fungus, Candida albicans, which causes thrush; or if it is due to infection by a small parasite, the size of the point of a pin, called Trichomonas vaginalis. Usually infection with either of these organisms causes an irritating vaginal discharge, but occasionally it does not. The doctor can only determine the actual cause of the vaginal discharge by examining a smear taken from the vagina with a cotton-wool swab. He looks at this under a microscope, and is then able to prescribe the appropriate treatment.

VARICOSE VEINS

Pregnancy provokes the appearance of varicose veins in the legs of women who are predisposed to them. The veins may appear at any time during pregnancy, but on the whole tend to enlarge and become more obvious in the later months. They may appear either as enlarged, worm-like tubes beneath the skin, or as spider varicosities around the ankles and behind the knees. The legs feel heavy, look ugly and may be painful or swollen. Most of the veins disappear once the baby is born, which is why doctors do not recommend surgical treatment in pregnancy. Some remain, however, to enlarge in subsequent pregnancies. Treatment is to keep the feet up as much as possible, and certainly to sit with the feet down as little as possible. As well as this, well-fitting supportive stockings, which are today indistinguishable from normal nylon stockings, should be put on each morning before the expectant mother puts her feet out of bed.

VITAMIN AND MINERAL SUPPLEMENTS

It is the habit of doctors, encouraged by the beautiful advertisements which appear in medical journals, to insist that all pregnant women receive tablets of vitamin and mineral 'supplements'. This habit is approved by convention, and the majority of women (at least in the U.S.A.) would feel that their doctor was being rather incompetent if he failed to prescribe a 'pregnancy pill'. The pregnant dietary supplementary pills often contain a multitude of minerals (for some of which it is admitted that no use has been found) and a variety of vitamins. These pills are swallowed with fair regularity by pregnant women, and I suspect in most cases the contained minerals and vitamins emerge from the other end unaltered, to join the vast concentration of the contents of swallowed pills and potions in the sewage. The question which has to be answered in the affluent countries, and particularly amongst the more affluent citizens in these countries, is: 'Are the pregnancy dietary supplements necessary?' Would not the money expended be better spent on some other natural foods? The answer must be a qualified 'Yes'! The great majority of women do not need pregnancy supplements provided they eat a reasonable diet. At the most they need to take each day a single pill containing iron. The 'submerged' 10 per cent of poor women in the affluent societies and the 90 per cent in the developing countries do need supplements, particularly of iron, but even more they need additional protein. These people are the very ones who all too often receive little antenatal care, usually get inadequate food, and most often receive no dietary supplementary pills in pregnancy. Their need is great; that of their affluent sisters is minimal.

The expectant mother should eat a balanced diet; she should obtain proper antenatal care; she should have the haemoglobin concentration of her blood tested, as described previously; and she should be given a prescription for a tablet containing an iron salt (and it does not matter which iron salt). She should take one of these tablets each day from about the 14th week of pregnancy, but if she happens to miss a couple of days, it does not matter much.

There has been some discussion recently about whether pregnant women should be given a particular vitamin called folic acid. It is called 'folic' acid because the vitamin was first found in the leaves of green vegetables, and *folium* is a leaf in Latin. This vitamin is needed for the growth of cells, and since little is stored in the body, a steady intake is required. In pregnancy the demand increases considerably, particularly in the last 10 weeks, and the level of folic acid in the mother's blood tends to fall. If the diet contains green or yellow leafy vegetables, lightly cooked using only a small amount of water, there is generally no need for additional folic acid tablets. But because the baby demands and takes so much folic acid from the mother, it may be wise to give supplements to the mother who is carrying twins. The dose she needs is very small, and the vitamin is only needed after the 30th week of pregnancy. The vitamin should only be taken after discussing the matter with the doctor.

What then is the situation regarding vitamin and mineral pills in pregnancy? Beyond taking a single iron tablet each day, and in special cases taking a folic acid tablet, the pregnant woman in an affluent society, who is not poor, does not require to take the vitamin and mineral pills so attractively displayed and bottled by enterprising pharmaceutical companies.

WEIGHT GAIN

It is quite obvious that women put on weight during pregnancy. The question to be answered is how much is permissible. Until very recently weight gain was restricted very considerably, as obstetricians believed that there was a close relationship between weight gain and the onset of 'toxaemia of pregnancy'. Whilst there is a relationship, it is now known that it is by no means as close as was previously thought. The rigid restriction on weight gain was especially propagated by American obstetricians, possibly because as a race Americans eat too much. At all events, women were bullied, frightened and indoctrinated into believing that a weight gain in pregnancy of more than 8 kg., or 18 lb., was dangerous, and in trying to restrict their weight gain to below this figure, many women had a miserable and anxious pregnancy. Today, it is known that this attitude was unnecessarily restrictive, and much more latitude can be allowed.

To appreciate how much weight gain is normal, it is helpful to analyse the various things which increase the expectant mother's weight in pregnancy. Obviously, the fetus, the placenta and the liquid in which the fetus lives all contribute. Equally obvious is the increased weight of the uterus and the breasts. Not quite so obvious is the fact that the increased volume of blood, which circulates in an expectant mother's arteries and veins, adds to the weight gain.

Two other factors are involved. The first is the increased deposition of fat in the mother's tissues. In part this is caused by the conversion of excess carbohydrate eaten in the diet, but in part is a normal event caused by the hormones of pregnancy. The amount of fat deposited varies very considerably. but averages 2.000 g.. or 4½ lb. It is believed that evolution of man led to this deposition of fat in pregnancy, so that the mother had extra energy stored which might later be needed for the care and feeding of her baby. Finally, and again because of the hormones of pregnancy, water is retained in the body. Again the amount varies, but about 4 litres, or 6¾ pints, is retained, half of it in the last 10 weeks of pregnancy.

It is possible to make a table showing how the various factors lead to weight gain in pregnancy:

Fetus, placenta and amniotic liquid		4400 g.	(10 lb. 0 oz.)
Uterus and breasts		1100 g.	(2 lb. 7 oz.)
Blood volume increase		1000 g.	(2 lb. 4 oz.)
Fat deposited	up to	2000 g.	(4 lb. 7 oz.)
Water retained	up to	4000 g.	(8 lb. 14 oz.)
		12.5 kg.	(28 lb. 0 oz.)

As can be seen, a total of 12.5 kg., or 28 lb., is a normal weight gain in pregnancy. Because of this, the doctors who restricted severely the patient's weight gain were being unnecessarily harsh.

The weight gain is not spread equally throughout pregnancy. After the 20th week, the fetus gains weight more rapidly, fat is deposited in greater amounts, and fluid is retained more readily. In fact, the expectation is that in the first 20 weeks a weight gain of 3.5 kg., or 8 lb., will occur, and in the last 20 weeks a weight gain of 9 kg., or 20 lb., can be considered normal. Of course, there are individual variations. The expectant mother who is underweight for her height may be encouraged to put on more weight, and the overweight mother will be firmly told not to put on so much weight.

More important than overall weight gain is the weekly gain in the last 20 weeks of pregnancy. A weight gain of more than 1 kg. (2 lb.) a week is suggestive of excess fat or fluid retention. This may be the first sign of 'toxaemia of pregnancy', so that the expectant mother should *avoid gaining more than 0.5 kg., or 1 lb., a week in the last 20 weeks of pregnancy.*

A final point, if an expectant mother gains more than 16 kg., or 35 lb., in pregnancy, she will find it almost impossible to loose the extra weight. Her clothes will not fit, her sylph-like figure will be a memory, and perhaps her husband will object. And that wouldn't do!

CHAPTER 12

Childbirth without pain

In the year 1847 in the city of Edinburgh, in the dining-room of a house in Queen Street, three respectable physicians sat sniffing the contents of various bottles. The bottles contained mixtures of chemicals which were said to cause loss of consciousness. They had spent many evenings in this pursuit, sniffing and recording their observations. On a cold, wet evening in November, the group led by James Young Simpson gathered as usual. One of the mixtures that night was a rather pleasant, sweet-smelling fluid. After one large whiff each, the three men became strangely excited and gay; after two, they all became sleepy; and after a third large inhalation, they lay sprawled on the floor, only awaking after a few minutes. In this way the anaesthetic qualities of chloroform were discovered. It was clear to Dr. Simpson that chloroform could help to relieve the pain of women in labour–for at that time no pain-relief of any kind was given, and as no patient received antenatal care, labours were often difficult, painful and dangerous. But when Simpson announced, in a paper published in the Monthly Journal of Medical Science, that chloroform could be used to relieve the pains of childbirth, he was criticised vehemently, attacked in print and from the pulpit by clergy and leaders of the public, as well as by many members of the medical profession. The use of chloroform was against God's Will, they cried, for was it not written that because Eve tempted Adam to eat the forbidden fruit, a curse was laid upon her that 'in sorrow would she bring forth her children'? If the pain and sorrow were reduced, it was irreligious. To this Simpson replied that in the Bible the first reported surgical operation had been performed under anaesthesia. The Lord God had caused 'a deep sleep to fall upon Adam; and he slept; and He took one of his ribs, and closed the flesh thereof'. Simpson was told by an American that to give chloroform was to interfere with nature, since the pains of childbirth were a natural function. Simpson agreed but asked, 'Is not walking also a natural function? And who would think of never setting aside or superseding this natural function. If you were travelling from Philadelphia to Baltimore, would you insist on walking the distance by foot simply because walking is man's natural method of locomotion?' An Irish woman visiting Scotland attacked him by saying. 'How unnatural it is for you doctors in Edinburgh to take away the pains of your patients when in labour'. His reply was, 'Madam, how unnatural it is for you to have swum over from Ireland to Scotland against wind and tides on a steamboat'.

Most of the objections were from the clergy; to each Simpson had an answer, and little by little his opponents were silenced, particularly as women appeared to approve of his attempt, in his own words, 'to alleviate human suffering, as well as preserve human life'. The cachet of approval was put upon his method when Queen Victoria was given inhalations of chloroform during the birth of her eighth child. Simpson was vindicated, and when he was later knighted, as Sir James Simpson, the opposition was in disorder. Yet to some extent, although they did not know it, they were partly right. Chloroform, although sweet-smelling, quick-acting and not irritating to breathe, is not a safe anaesthetic, because it may damage the liver. Consequently it is no longer used in obstetric practice.

No one would now deny that women should have the discomfort of childbirth relieved, and countless methods have been introduced in the past. Some were dangerous to the mother, some to the child; but today a reasonable approach has been made, and women need no longer fear the pain of childbirth. There are very real dangers though if the sedation is pushed too far, and the doctors have to find out the point at which adequate sedation and analgesia (that is, pain-relief without unconsciousness) can be given without risk to the mother or baby. It is unfair to promise a mother that all discomfort can be relieved, but it is equally callous for a doctor to allow his patient to suffer unduly, or to permit the nurses, who are so much closer to the patient during most of labour, to appear indifferent to her discomfort or perhaps even to relish it. Luckily only a few of these midwives remain, and today the training of a nurse-midwife includes instruction in analgesia.

In the U.S.A., particularly, women are given large quantities of analgesics, and are often delivered under anaesthesia for no reason other than relieving pain. It has been felt by some obstetricians that the degree of anaesthesia is too deep, that less anaesthetic could be given so that pain was relieved but labour was more natural, and the mother had the joy of seeing the birth of her baby. It has also been found that the mother who knows what will happen during labour, who knows how the baby descends through the birth-canal and is born, and who knows what is expected of her, requires far less sedation in labour. This observation led the Russians initially, and subsequently the French, to offer a system of instruction to pregnant women which reduces the need for analgesics, and in fact eliminates them altogether in 45 per cent of women in labour. This method is called 'Psychoprophylaxis'.

PSYCHOPROPHYLAXIS

In many cultures pregnancy and childbirth are considered shameful matters, to be hidden from view and not discussed. As a consequence of this, many women have no idea what happens in childbirth, and how a large baby can be born through what appears to be a small hole. Strangely, even today, some pregnant women believe, until told otherwise, that the baby is born through the umbilicus. Because childbirth is not discussed, many women pregnant for the first time only learn of its processes from equally-ill-informed friends and older women, who all too readily tell the young girl of the 'terrible time I had before the doctor cut out the baby', and of the pain, agony and danger of childbirth. According to the Russians, these snippets of misinformation sink deep into the memory of the pregnant woman, and a 'conditioned reflex' occurs. Because of this reflex, every time the girl thinks of childbirth, a mental image of pain, suffering, danger of death and fear is conjured up, so that a woman enters labour anxious and tense. Psychoprophylaxis seeks to eliminate this 'conditioned reflex', and replace the image of fear, anxiety and tenseness by one in which childbirth is known to be a normal event. It also seeks to alter the brain's appreciation of pain, and convert it into a sensation of discomfort which can be relieved by muscular activity.

The psychoprophylactic method depends on the belief that 'conditioned reflexes' can be changed by training, because they are not built into the person's personality, but arise because of the person's response (or conditioning) to outside events.

It is known that pain is a relative thing. Pain is felt in a different way at different times. A hypnotized person, although awake, feels no pain; a soldier in the field, cold, deserted, hungry and wounded, may feel considerably more pain from his wound than he would if he were warm, rescued and being looked after by a sympathetic nurse. The pain of a dentist's drill varies depending on how much confidence the person has in her dentist, and how she herself feels. And, of course, each person has her own threshold above which pain is felt: the stoic woman feels little pain; the anxious, nervous person, given the same degree of pain, will feel a lot.

These facts are utilized in the psychoprophylactic method. The brain of every person is thought to have a special threshold below which no pain is felt. The normal, everyday, potentially painful stimuli which occur are not interpreted as pain because they fall below the threshold at which pain is felt. But the threshold can be reduced by conditions such as fear, emotional upset, shock, hunger and cold. In these conditions, stimuli which are normally not painful cross the lowered pain threshold and are felt as pain. Psychoprophylaxis seeks to raise the pain threshold by explanation of the processes of labour. And by the exercises which are taught seeks to change the interpretation by the patient's mind of any painful sensations which get over the threshold. By changing pain to muscular activity, the patient actively participates in the childbirth.

Training takes place along two main lines. Firstly, the fear of labour is reduced or eliminated by a series of talks in which the mother is told how conception occurs, how the fetus grows, what happens in childbirth, and how she can help by learning breathing techniques. Secondly, she is taught certain exercises, which are thought to improve her muscular control.

The breathing exercises, which are taught in the second half of pregnancy, are of three kinds. The first two are for use in the first stage of labour, and the third for helping to expel the baby from the mother's birth-canal in the second stage of labour.

The breathing exercises for the first stage of labour are to learn slow quiet breathing using the rib muscles, and not the diaphragm. The patient learns by demonstration and by reiteration that the onset of a contraction of her womb is a signal for her to start her learnt breathing pattern. In this way she learns that a contraction is a signal for breathing activity, rather than pain. In the late first stage, when the contractions are stronger, she learns that a breathing pattern of quick, shallow breathing interspersed with breath blown out at intervals helps considerably, especially if she combines the breathing with 'effleurage'. This is a light stroking movement of the fingers over the abdomen.

In the second stage of labour the pattern of breathing changes again. The expectant mother now takes deep breaths, which steady her diaphragm against the upper part of her uterus. This is followed by a contraction of her chest and upper abdominal muscles, which form a girdle around the uterus adding its pressure effects to those of the uterine contractions. In the first stage of labour, she should lie on one side or the other, whilst in the second stage she lies on her back, reclining upon pillows beneath her head and shoulders.

As well as breathing exercises, many supporters of psycho-prophylaxis believe that certain exercises encourage muscular control. For a muscular contraction to occur, the message (or stimulus) must travel from the brain to the muscle, and when one muscle contracts, others have to relax. Muscles which act in this way are called voluntary muscles, as they are under the control of the mind. (Not all muscles are voluntary; some, like those of the uterus and the heart, are involuntary and contract independently of the person's wishes.) To accomplish the delivery of her baby through her vulva in the second stage of labour with the greatest ease, the mother has to contract her abdominal muscles in time with the uterine contractions, and simultaneously relax the muscles which support her vagina and perineum. The exercises learnt in 'relaxation classes' help her to do this.

Throughout the training period, the mother learns that the breathing exercises and exercises for 'neuro-muscular' control will help her during labour, but she is told that if she finds she requires pain-killing drugs, these will be given readily, and she must not feel a sense of failure about needing them. It has been found that the best results are obtained if the patient is confident in her knowledge of the processes of labour, if she constantly receives support and encouragement from those attending her, and if she is told from time to time of her progress.

ANALGESICS AND SEDATIVES

Using psychoprophylactic methods, about 45 per cent of women require no sedation or analgesics, 45 per cent require some sedation, and 10 per cent are not helped by the method. Psychoprophylaxis demands the co-operation of the patient or it fails, and its impact outside Russia and France is not great. It is right that women in labour should be offered drugs which will help them. In early labour the uterine contractions are not painful, and analgesics (or 'pain-killers') are not required, but apprehensive women may welcome a sedative. The two main groups are the barbiturates and the tranquillizers. Barbiturates are sedative drugs derived from barbituric acid, and the derivative may be effective for a long, a medium or a short time. Usually a short- or medium-acting drug is chosen. These drugs are avoided when labour is well established, as they have unpredictable effects, and may slightly reduce the newborn baby's ability to breathe properly.

Perhaps more useful are the tranquillizers. Many different tranquillizers have been used in labour, but most obstetricians agree that promazine is one of the best. It is usually given by injection into a muscle when labour is established, and gives the mother a warm, 'woozy' feeling.

When labour is really under way, and the contractions are strong, many women want an analgesic which will reduce the painful sensations. In pride of place is pethidine (called meperidine in the U.S.A.). Pethidine is given by injection into a muscle, usually in the thigh, and dulls pain in about 20 minutes, the effect lasting from two to five hours, so that several injections may be needed during the course of labour. It has been given to many thousands of women in labour, with safety and with effectiveness.

ANAESTHETICS

Towards the end of the first stage of labour and in the second stage, the mother may require further help to reduce the discomfort. Two anaesthetics are available for this. In both cases the patient holds a mask over her face and breathes deeply during a uterine contraction. The drug in the gas mixture dulls the pain, and once the contraction has ceased, the mother puts the mask on one side. The two anaesthetic mixtures are 'gas and oxygen' and 'Trilene'. There is little to choose between them. 'Gas' (really nitrous oxide) is mixed in a special machine with oxygen, so that there is never less than 30 per cent of oxygen in the mixture. The patient breathes this mixture through a tube and face-mask. 'Trilene' is a sweet-smelling, blue liquid, which vapourizes into a gas when air is passed over it. Trilene is placed in a small box-like inhaler, and this is connected by a rubber tube to a face-mask. When the patient breathes in through the tube, air passes over the Trilene and some vapour is taken up. As a contraction starts, the mother breathes in, and inhales Trilene vapour which dulls her pain. Between contractions she puts the mask to one side. Not every woman can use Trilene.

Epidural anaesthesia

The backbone is made up of separate vertebrae, and protects the spinal cord, which extends as far down as the pelvis through a hole in each vertebra. The spinal cord is made up of millions of nerve fibres, and is linked to all parts of the body. Impulses are constantly passing from all parts of the body to the brain along the spinal cord, and out again from the brain to all parts of the body. A substantial number of the nerves relay to the brain sensations received by the various parts of the body, such as feelings of cold, heat or pain. The nerves relaying these sensations are called sensory nerve fibres, and they pass along different routes from the nerve fibres which bring messages from the brain to the muscles and other structures. Since many of these fibres make the muscles contract, or move, they are called motor fibres. If it were possible to anaesthetize, or numb, the sensory fibres from the uterus without also anaesthetizing the motor fibres to the uterus, labour could be made painless. Luckily this can be done safely, provided the anaesthetist is an expert.

The spinal cord is surrounded by a glistening envelope (called the dura) for all of its length, and the envelope contains a fluid. Between the envelope and the bony hole in the vertebrae is a space, through which nerves pass from the spinal cord on their way to and from the structures of the body (Fig. **12/1**). The anaesthetist inserts a thin needle through the muscles of the mother's back, and with great care gets the tip to lie in the space between the dura and the bone–this is the epidural space. He pushes a fine polythene tube through

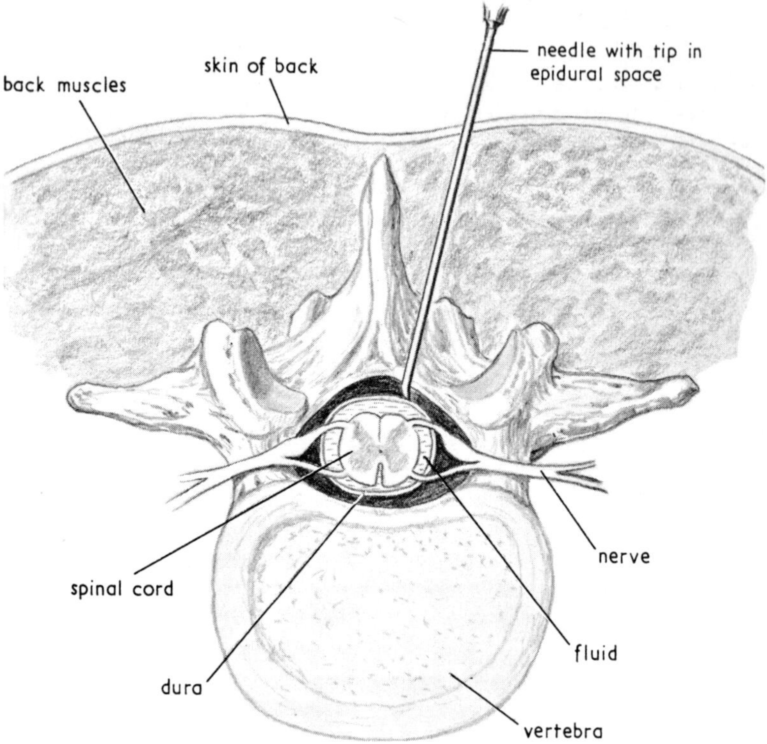

FIG 12/1. Epidural anaethesia

the needle so that it is in the space, and then withdraws the needle, leaving the polythene tube in the space. He can now give a local anaesthetic into the epidural space, and, if needs be, keep 'topping' it up when the anaesthetic effect begins to wear off. Epidural anaesthesia is very effective, as all pain goes but the patient remains conscious and can co-operate. However, it is not suitable for every woman, and many more will not require it. But in certain patients it is a splendid anaesthetic.

Pudendal or perineal nerve block

The final phase of labour, when the baby's head begins to stretch the tissues around the vulva, can be quite painful, especially in a first labour. Many doctors believe that the mother can be made more comfortable by giving her a local anaesthetic injection into the tissues, so that the 'bursting feeling' is eliminated. This is now quite usual, and apart from a tiny prick, is painless. More important, the 'bursting' pain in the vulva disappears very quickly after the injection.

'PAINLESS CHILDBIRTH'

Childbirth is rarely completely painless, but with good preparation in pregnancy, with the choice of sedatives, analgesics and anaesthetic agents now available, it can be made reasonably comfortable. When this occurs, the mother herself can help in the process of childbirth, and can have the joy of witnessing the birth of her baby.

CHAPTER 13

The three stages of labour

The process of childbirth is usually called 'labour'. The term is appropriate, for labour is a time of work. Considerable energy is expended in the contractions of the uterus. For this reason the pregnant woman is in ways like an athlete. If she has had proper training during pregnancy, so that she knows what to expect and what to do in labour; if she is in good physical condition; if her mental attitude to labour is good, the process of childbirth is relatively easy. One of the objectives of good antenatal care is to enable her to reach this peak of fitness at the time labour is due.

Before we consider the process of labour from the viewpoint of the expectant mother, it is helpful to consider what happens in labour. With the aid of diagrams, it will be shown how the baby is expelled from its heat-controlled capsule, to journey down the dark curved birth-canal, and to be pushed out into a world where it has to use many functions for which it had no need while in the uterus. It has to obtain its oxygen from the atmosphere, not from its mother's blood. It has to get rid of its own waste products. It can no longer depend upon its placenta to act as a liver and a kidney. It has to obtain food instead of depending on the transfer across the placenta of required foodstuffs from the mother's blood to its own blood. In all these functions, the newborn baby succeeds admirably. However, the more normal the process of childbirth, the easier it is for the baby to adjust to independent life.

THE LAST FEW DAYS OF PREGNANCY

In late pregnancy, just before the onset of labour, the baby has grown to an average weight of 3,300 gm. ($7\frac{1}{2}$ lb.), and is 50 cm. (20 in.) long. It has occupied more and more space in the amniotic sac, and the amount of amniotic fluid has been reduced from a maximum volume of 1,000 ml. ($1\frac{3}{4}$ pints) at 36 weeks' gestation, to about 600 ml. (1 pint) at 40 weeks' gestation, or 'term'. If it is a first pregnancy, the baby's head is likely to have settled into the mother's pelvis. The uterus is becoming increasingly sensitive to stimuli, and increasingly active. The cervix is soft, has shortened in length, and is likely to have begun to open a bit, usually about 1 to 2 finger-breadths. If a doctor performs a pelvic examination at this stage, he will feel the 'bag of waters', which is the inexact term used for the amniotic sac, and in it he can feel the baby's head. If he could see the baby, he would find in more than three-quarters of cases that its face was looking towards the mother's right or left hip bone (Fig. **13/1**).

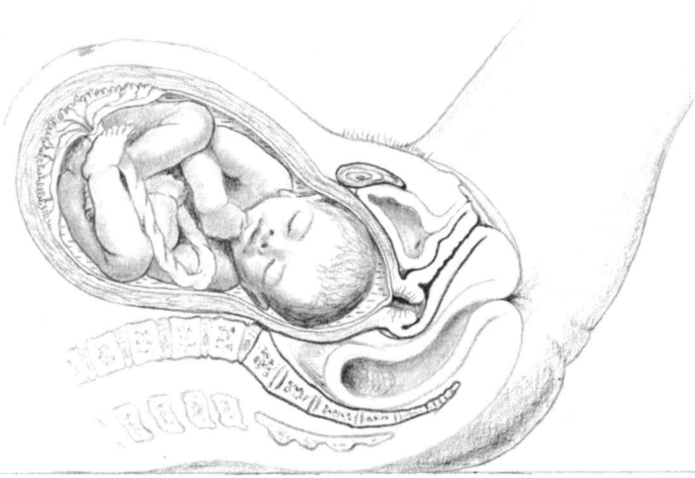

FIG. 13/1. The baby in late pregnancy. Its head is 'fixed' in the mother's pelvis and it 'looks' towards one hip bone. The cervix is soft but not yet drawn up

THE FIRST STAGE OF LABOUR

For reasons which are quite unknown, at a specific point in time labour starts. The uterine contractions initially are not very strong, and only occur at long intervals. However, with the passage of time, they become stronger and more frequent. This phase of labour does not distress the patient unduly, and is called the quiet phase. It lasts an average of 9 hours in a first labour, and 4 hours in subsequent labours.

With each contraction, the muscle fibres of the uterus shorten a tiny fraction, so that a pull is exerted on the cervix, which is the weakest part. This is because the muscle is thickest in the upper part of the uterus, and becomes less thick in the lower part. The cervix has only 10 per cent of muscle.

The pull on the cervix firstly shortens it until it no longer hangs down into the vagina like a cuff, but is drawn up flush. Doctors call this 'cervical effacement'. The pull then opens the cervix, and it slowly opens wider and wider. This the doctors call 'cervical dilatation', and patients may hear nurses or doctors saying that the cervix is so many finger-breadths, or so many centimetres dilated. The quiet phase of labour usually lasts until the cervix is 2 to 3 finger-breadths (or 4 to 5 centimetres) dilated. Three fingers, or 5 centimetres, means that the cervix is half-way to its complete opening, which doctors call 'full dilatation'.

During the quiet phase, the baby's head flexes more so that it tucks in its chin, and the head moves more deeply into the pelvis. This can be seen in the illustration. It will be noted that the 'bag of waters' is still intact (Fig. **13/2**). The end of the quiet phase is heralded by a change in the character of the uterine contractions. They become stronger and more frequent, and the expectant mother may request drugs to reduce the discomfort. The cervix continues to dilate, and the baby is pushed further into the pelvis, where it may cause pressure on the bladder and back-passage (Fig. **13/3**). As the dilatation of the cervix becomes nearly complete, the contractions of the uterus are quite strong, but the degree of discomfort felt by the patient will depend on the adequacy of her preparation for labour, and on her attitude to labour. When the cervix is fully dilated, the uterus and vagina together form a curved passage, along which the baby can pass aided by uterine contractions and the mother's additional use of her abdominal muscles.

The period of time from the onset of labour to the full dilatation of the cervix is called the *first stage of labour*. It lasts, on an average, 13 hours in a first labour, and 7 hours in a subsequent labour, although, of course, the duration of the first stage varies very considerably between different expectant mothers.

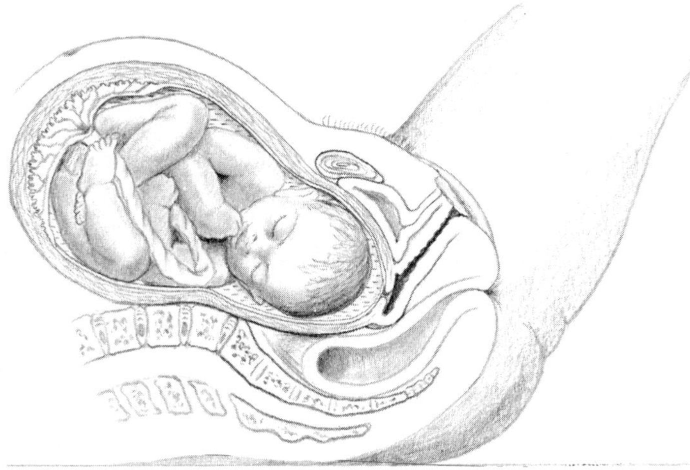

FIG. 13/2. The baby in early labour. Note how it has tucked its chin well in. The cervix has been drawn up, and the bag of waters is still intact

FIG. 13/3. Late in the first stage of labour. The cervix has almost completely opened and the bag of waters bulges in front of the head

THE SECOND STAGE OF LABOUR

The second stage of labour is the time when the mother-to-be has to help. In the first stage she helps most by relaxing during contractions, and by reading, talking, listening to the radio or watching television. In the second stage she has work to do. She has to aid in the expulsion of the baby from the birth-canal, which is formed from the uterus and the vagina. The second stage usually lasts less than 1½ hours, extending in time from the full dilatation of the cervix to the birth of the baby. If the second stage lasts longer than 1½ hours, the attending doctor usually helps the birth by forceps (see Chapter 17). The beginning of the second stage is announced frequently by the bursting of the 'bag of waters', with a resulting gush of fluid from the vagina. The bursting of the 'bag of waters', called by doctors 'rupture of the membranes', may occur much earlier in labour, or occasionally not until the baby is ready to be born. Usually, however, it occurs at the very end of the first stage of labour.

At the same time the expectant mother gets the urge to push. This is caused by the pressure of the baby's head on the tissues in the middle of the pelvis. A message is sent to the brain, which makes the mother want to fix her diaphragm, and contract her abdominal muscles to push her baby out into the world. The baby is therefore pushed downwards, and because of the shape of the muscles which stretch across the pelvis, its head turns so that it comes to look backwards (Fig. **13/5**). Evolution has caused this, for when man expanded his brain and developed a round skull, he made childbirth more difficult. The widest diameter at the entrance to the bony pelvis is the one stretching across it between the hip bones, and the baby adjusts so that the long diameter of its head (that from the forehead backwards) fits into this. In the lower part of the pelvis, the longest diameter is from before backwards, and the baby's head rotates to fit this so that its face now looks backward towards the mother's back.

With each contraction of the uterus, and aided by the mother's 'pushing' efforts, the baby's head moves nearer the vulval cleft. Soon the top of its head can be seen by the doctor who will deliver the baby. The head advances a bit with each contraction, and retreats a bit between contractions, but overall the advance continues, more

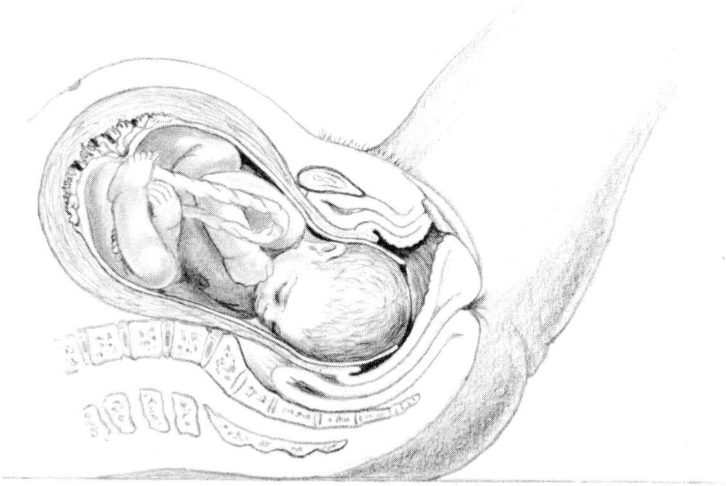

FIG. 13/4. The early part of the second stage of labour. The child's head is beginning to turn so that it faces towards its mother's back. The bag of waters has 'broken'. The mother feels pressure on her bladder and rectum, and she has the desire to push

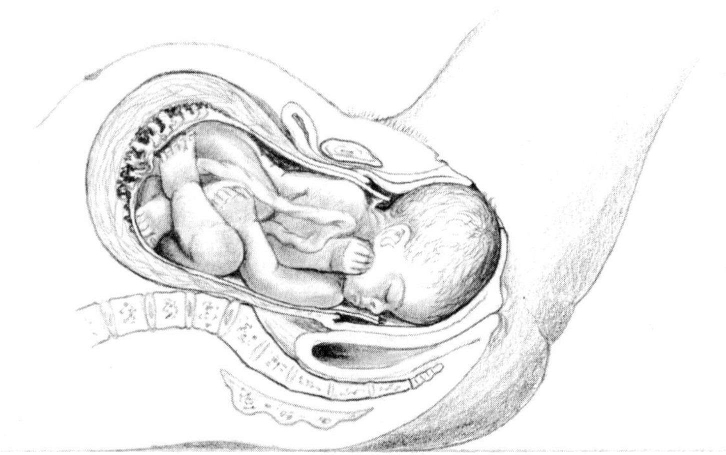

FIG. 13/5. Late second stage. Labour is nearly over. The baby's head appears at the vulva, and the shoulders are turning to fit into the bones of the pelvis. The face is turned completely towards the mother's back. The mother's perineum is being stretched

and more of the head becoming visible. The mother is working very hard during this time, her pulse rises, she sweats from the effort, and between contractions she rests, dozing and obtaining energy for the next effort. And despite this, it is said that women are the 'weaker sex'! Finally, the head stretches the vaginal entrance and the tissues between it and the back-passage (or anus). This area is called the perineum, and it becomes tightly stretched over the baby's head which bulges through it. This is quaintly called 'crowning of the head'. At this point the doctor may inject a local anaesthetic into the tissues of the vulva, if he has not done so already. This prevents the mother from the pain of stretching of the tissues, which many say feels as if their bottom was about to burst. They also say it resembles the feeling of trying to open the bowels after being constipated for a month! The next contraction pushes the baby down further, and the head sweeps over the vulval tissues, the forehead, the eyes, the nose, the mouth and the chin appearing successively (Fig. **13/6**).

The delivery of the baby's head can be seen in the series of drawings (Fig. **13/7**), and it can be noted that once the head is born, it turns back to face the mother's hips. This has been arranged by

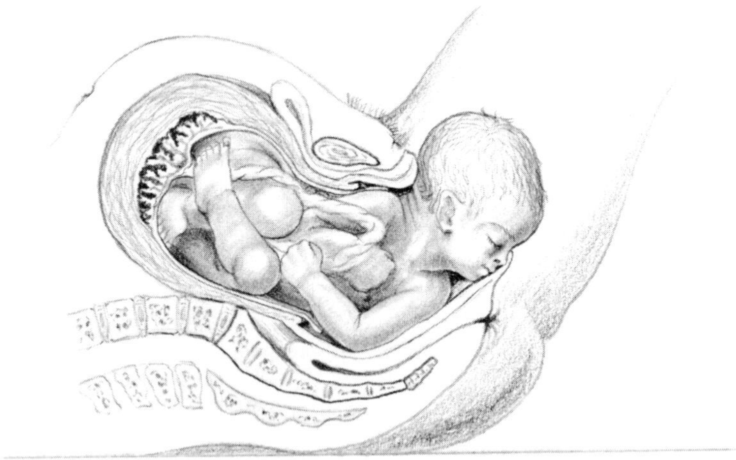

FIG. 13/6. The baby's head is being born, emerging from the vagina and sweeping the perineum backwards

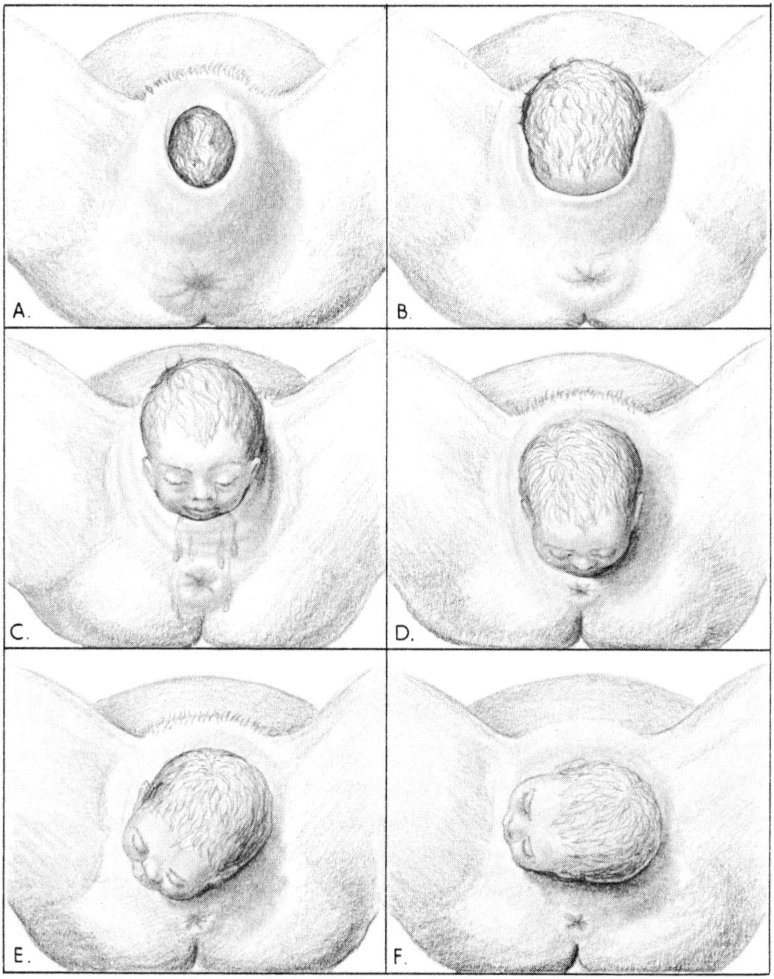

FIG. 13/7. The birth of the baby's head as seen by the doctor

evolution so that the shoulders of the baby and the rest of its body can slip out of the birth-canal easily. The baby is born! The mother, no longer expectant, looks delightedly at her baby, and as its first cry echoes, she fondles it and then relaxes and sleeps momentarily.

THE THIRD STAGE OF LABOUR

Little more remains but to wait for the expulsion of the placenta, or afterbirth, so-called for obvious reasons. This has separated from its attachment to the wall of the uterus as the baby was born. The doctor either awaits its expulsion or, as is more usual today, aids its rapid removal by giving an injection of a drug which makes the uterus contract firmly. This, of course, reduces the blood lost by the mother, which is desirable.

CHAPTER 14

What to expect in labour

The mechanical processes which lead to the birth of the baby need to be understood by the expectant mother, so that she may have insight into what happens and what is expected of her. But she also needs to know what happens to her and what she is to do.

LATE PREGNANCY AND PRELABOUR

In the last weeks of pregnancy, the baby is settling into its final position preparatory to birth. In the majority of first pregnancies the baby's head has settled into the pelvis and is exerting pressure on the pelvis, the rectum and the bladder. Varicose veins become more obvious as the blood returning from the legs is dammed back; backache is more common; frequency of urination usual. The expectant mother, too, is becoming impatient. She wants to see and fondle the baby she has nurtured all these weeks. Sleep is less sound, and on hot nights sweating may be a problem. It is quite proper for the expectant mother to ask her doctor for sleeping tablets to help 'tide' her over these last few weeks; but most women adjust to the disturbed nights, and rest during the day to make up for it.

False labour

In these weeks, the uterus is increasingly sensitive, and the painless contractions which have been felt in the preceding weeks become more frequent. Painful contractions may also occur, usually at night and at irregular intervals. This is 'false labour', but it may be mistaken for the onset of true labour, and many an expectant mother has been admitted to hospital, only to be discharged home the next day. The difference between false and true labour is that the contractions in false labour are irregular in duration, occur at irregular intervals, and rather than increasing in intensity (or strength) as time passes, diminish in intensity after a few hours and then disappear altogether. Often they occur at night, and are usually felt in the lower abdomen and back. This is in contrast to true labour, in which there is an increasing frequency and intensity of contractions, which develop an almost predictable regularity as time progresses. But no mother should be ashamed of having gone into hospital in false labour, as sometimes the two types are most difficult to differentiate.

What to take into hospital

By this time the expectant mother will have prepared the things which she will require in hospital, and will often have a bag packed in readiness. What she needs depends to some extent on her own desires and local custom. In general the bag should contain the following:

Nightdress or pyjamas (2 or 3 sets). Many women prefer pyjamas, and wear the top only. In many ways pyjamas are more convenient than nightdresses, particularly if the mother is going to breast feed. A few hospitals, regrettably, insist that the patient wear a hospital gown. This is generally ugly. The practice is disappearing, and the sooner it goes, the better.

Brassières. Two nursing brassières are usually required.

Bed jacket

Dressing gown. This is essential as 'early ambulation' is now normal, and patients are usually up and about within 24 to 48 hours of childbirth.

Bedroom slippers

Sanitary belt. Sanitary pads are usually supplied by the hospital, but some hospitals ask the patient to supply her own, and to bring them in before labour so that they may be sterilized.

Handkerchiefs or tissues

Toothpaste, toothbrush, toilet soap, washing flannel, nail brush, hairbrush, comb, hand mirror, cosmetics, perfume, talcum powder. Beauty may be in the eye of the beholder, and the new mother has every right to feel and be beautiful. But artifacts help in our society, and why not?

Writing paper, envelopes, stamps and a pen. It is surprising how many letters need to be written once the baby is born.

Books. The lying-in period is a time of rest, interspersed with moments of activity. Books fill in the time, although portable television sets are regrettably replacing them.

Baby clothes. A set for dressing the baby on discharge from hospital. Hospitals usually supply nightgowns and napkins (diapers) for the hospital period.

THE ONSET OF LABOUR

The onset of true labour is announced by one or more of the following three signs:

(1) The onset of regular, rhythmic uterine contractions, which may be painful.

(2) The passage of a small amount of blood-tinged, sticky mucus from the vagina (the 'show').

(3) The 'gushing' of liquid from the vagina. This is due to rupture of the membranes which form the amniotic sac.

Regular painful contractions

If false labour has been experienced in the last weeks of pregnancy, the patient may be able to detect a change in the character of the contractions when true labour starts. If no false labour has been experienced, the patient will be able to determine if this is indeed true labour from the character of the contractions. The contractions of true labour initially last about 30 seconds, and occur at regular intervals of about 15 to 20 minutes. During the contraction, the uterus can be felt to become hard, and some degree of pain is felt, either only in the small of the back, or, as labour progresses, radiating from the flanks into the abdomen. In fact, as a rule the less backache there is, the more efficient is the labour. The pain begins as a small 'twinge', it increases to a peak, and diminishes to fade away entirely. In the opinion of many women, it is like a severe menstrual cramp.

As labour progresses, the duration of the contraction extends from 30 seconds to 90 seconds; the interval between contractions diminishes from 20 minutes to 3 or 5 minutes, and the intensity of the contraction increases, so that the expectant mother may ask for pain-reducing drugs.

In general, the patient should go into hospital when the contractions are regular and are recurring at about 10 minute intervals, but of course this is only 'in general', and individuals may feel the need to go into hospital earlier or later.

The 'show'

The discharge of blood-stained mucus precedes or accompanies the onset of painful contractions as often as it follows them. What has happened is that the 'plug' of mucus which has filled the cervical canal from early pregnancy is dislodged as the uterine contractions draw up (or 'efface') the cervix and begin to dilate it at the onset of labour. The discharge of the blood-stained mucus is called the 'show', and labour generally starts within 24 hours of its appearance.

Rupture of the membranes

In a few cases, labour is heralded by a sudden gush of liquid from the vagina. This occurs because the membranes of the amniotic sac, which lines the uterus and in which the baby has grown, suddenly rupture. This event may occur before term, or it may occur at term. In either event, the patient should go to the hospital without delay, so that she may be examined, as occasionally problems arise which need to be checked as soon as possible. In general, labour starts within a few hours of spontaneous rupture of the membranes. If labour has not started within 12 to 24 hours and the pregnancy is near term, the doctor will give an infusion of a drug called oxytocin, into an arm vein of the expectant mother, to hasten the onset of labour.

ADMISSION TO HOSPITAL

From time to time newspaper stories appear of women who failed to reach hospital in time, and the baby was born in the car, in a taxi, or perhaps on the front steps of the hospital. These occurrences are rare, and most expectant mothers get into hospital in good time.

For doctors and nurses a hospital is a familiar workplace; for many patients it is a strange and frightening place, where unbending people order the patient to do unpredictable things, and where everyone seems too busy to talk to her and to explain what is being done and why. This authoritarian, inhuman approach is fast going, and hospitals are becoming places in which *people* work to help other people. As childbirth is an essentially normal event, this humanist approach is even more important in a maternity hospital, and happily it is becoming much more common. One way in which the expectant mother can reduce her anxiety is to visit the hospital during pregnancy. Many hospital authorities co-operate in arranging these visits, when the patient can see the labour ward, or delivery floor, and the type of room, or ward, in which she will stay.

On admission in early labour, it is usually the practice for the patient to be examined by a doctor on the hospital staff or a nurse, who will then inform the patient's own doctor, depending on the custom and staff pattern of the particular hospital. The first thing which is done is to determine if labour is really under way, and how far advanced it is. This information is obtained from the patient's description of what has happened in the preceding few hours, aided if necessary by an abdominal examination of the position of the baby in the uterus. If labour is not far advanced, it is usual for the patient to change into a hospital gown and to get into bed, so that she may be 'prepared' for delivery. In the past this preparation was fairly complex: the patient had a hot bath, was given an enema, and the pubic and vulval hair was shaved. Today, the hot bath is replaced by a warm shower, if the patient feels she needs one. The enema is omitted, or replaced by the use of a small pill which is inserted into the back-passage, and induces a bowel motion with much less discomfort and distress than did the enema. The 'complete' shave is reduced to shaving the area of the perineum, the hair on the pubis merely being clipped short. The old method of a complete shave was uncomfortable (nurses are not very skilful with a safety razor), undignified, the patient feeling that she looked like a 'plucked chicken', and not really necessary unless an abdominal operation was anticipated.

When these preliminaries are over, the resident doctor usually reviews the patient's antenatal record if this is available, and checks that she is not suffering from any infectious disease such as a cold. He then examines a specimen of urine and takes the patient's blood pressure. Next he re-examines the abdomen to make sure that the baby is lying normally, and that the head or the breech is fitting into the expectant mother's pelvis. He may also wish to perform a pelvic examination so that he can make a full evaluation of the progress of labour. This examination is in no way different from the pelvic examination performed in pregnancy, except that increased precautions are taken to avoid infection. Whilst the doctor is cleaning his hands, the patient is placed on a sterile cloth and may put on leggings. The doctor cleans the vulval area with an antiseptic solution, and pours some obstetric antiseptic cream into the vagina. This not only prevents infection, but also renders the examination easier. During these examinations the doctor will be able to answer any questions which the patient may have.

THE FIRST STAGE OF LABOUR

The first stage of labour is the time during which the cervix must be drawn up and opened fully so that the birth-canal is established. It is a time when the expectant mother can actively do little to aid the delivery of her baby. It is a period of waiting intelligently, with the knowledge of the preparations for the birth of her child which are occurring within her body.

Since it is a period of waiting, more and more hospitals and obstetricians are coming to realize that during the first stage the patient requires to be in an atmosphere which is as home-like as possible, and only when the end of this stage is approaching does she need to be taken to the more antiseptic hospital-like surroundings of the delivery ward. To meet the needs of this new philosophy, hospitals are building (or converting other accommodation into) first stage areas, which contain individual rooms and a common-room, decorated pleasantly, furnished with comfortable chairs, and perhaps with a television set so that the patient may occupy her time more happily.

As has been noted, the patient who has insight into the processes of labour, and who has perhaps been to psychoprophylactic classes in pregnancy, is much better equipped to cope with the first stage of labour. At some time it is likely that the contractions will become uncomfortably strong. When this occurs, the expectant mother usually wishes to go to bed, and may request pain-reducing drugs, which are readily available. She will also be confined to bed if the membranes have ruptured or if any other complication has been detected. In the first stage the patient should not lie on her back on a hard bed. She should either recline propped up on pillows or lie on her side, as in this way she improves the flow of blood through the uterus, and provides more oxygen for her baby.

During the first stage of labour, she will not be permitted to eat any solid food, for the good reason that in labour food remains in the stomach and is not digested; and she may not be permitted to drink any fluids. Some doctors do permit their patients to drink tea, water or sweet drinks; others feel that all fluid should be given as an infusion into an arm vein.

THE SECOND STAGE

This is the stage of expulsion of the baby from the warm womb into the outside world. This is the period when the active aid of the mother is required to help her baby be born. It is a time of some discomfort, which is reduced by modern anaesthetic methods and by the injection of local anaesthetic into the tissues at the entrance of the vagina.

The help of the mother is needed. With each uterine contraction she takes in a big breath, filling her lungs with air. She then holds her breath, which makes her diaphragm rigid, and by contracting her lower chest and abdominal muscles, she pushes down, adding a further expulsive effort. Often she finds that she can get a better 'push' if she lifts her head and clasps her legs, drawing them up onto her abdomen. During a contraction she works hard, between contractions she relaxes completely. To dull the pain of the contraction, she may breathe 'gas and oxygen' from a machine, or another gas called 'Trilene'. The practice differs in different hospitals.

At last the baby's head appears, stretching the tissues of the perineum. Rather than allowing the perineum to tear jaggedly, as may happen, the doctor often makes a deliberate small cut with scissors. This is called an 'episiotomy'. It is easier to stitch, is much less painful if stitched properly (in fact using one technique it is virtually painless), and heals far better.

A final push 'crowns' the baby's head and the doctor now helps in delivering the baby. The expectant mother only pushes when she is asked to do so, instead panting quietly as the baby is slowly and gently born. The birth of the baby from 'crowning of the head' takes about 2 or 3 minutes, and many doctors give an injection at this time to expel the placenta more rapidly. But not all agree that this is necessary.

The baby is born, and lies between the mother's legs whilst its nose and throat are cleared of mucus. The cord which has been its lifeline for 40 weeks ceases to beat; it is tied and cut. The baby takes a breath and its first cry is heard by the mother, who is lying back relaxed. The doctor makes sure that the baby is normal–and over 97 per cent are–and then hands the baby to the mother, so that she may fondle and cuddle it whilst the afterbirth is being expelled.

Indeed, some doctors–and I am one of them–encourage the patient to witness the birth of her baby. If the expectant mother is propped up on pillows, she can see the baby being born once the head has been crowned, and can hold its waving hands whilst the buttocks are still emerging from her body.

THE THIRD STAGE

The third and final stage of labour is the time during which the placenta is expelled. It rarely lasts for more than 20 minutes, and is painless. Usually, today, the doctor assists the expulsion of the placenta by pressure upwards on the abdomen just above the pubic bone, and by gently pulling on the cut cord at the same time. A small amount of bleeding is usual during the third stage, but it is less than 300 ml. ($\frac{1}{2}$ pint) in most cases, particularly if the injection mentioned earlier has been given. The injection makes the uterus contract firmly, and the blood vessels which have supplied the placenta are squeezed tightly in the lattice of muscle fibres.

Labour is over. The episiotomy is stitched. The mother, no longer expectant but fulfilled, is washed and powdered. She relaxes and sometimes sleeps whilst the nurses check that the uterus is contracted, and about one hour after delivery she returns to her room in the lying-in ward. She is emotionally happy. She has done a unique and wonderful thing.

THE FATHER IN LABOUR

What of the father? It was his spermatozoon which fertilized the egg; it is he who has contributed half of the genes to the child. What is his place in labour? This depends greatly on custom and culture. In some tribal societies the man undergoes a mock labour, is pampered and cossetted during the time his wife, either alone or attended by a single female, delivers her child. In other societies, the man is excluded from the vicinity of the place where the woman has her baby, and is expected to ignore the whole episode, holding that it never happened.

In modern Western society, there is a trend to involve the father in the process of childbirth. He, as well as the mother, reads about the process of growth of the child in the uterus; he learns about the course of labour; together they are involved in the sequence of events leading up to childbirth. This approach has much to commend it. It culminates in the presence of the father during childbirth. In the first stage of labour he remains with his wife, so that in the unfamiliar surroundings of the hospital, she has someone whom she knows, loves and with whom she can share her experiences. An expectant mother should never be left alone in labour. This ideal is often difficult to achieve, and the presence of the father can be invaluable. In the second stage of labour, he sits by the head of the delivery bed, attending to his wife, encouraging her, being involved with her. Together they witness the birth of the baby, and together their emotional bonds are strengthened. In using this method for some years, I have observed its value repeatedly; and the look of joy on the faces of father and mother as together they help in the delivery of their child is wonderful.

The question which must be answered is, 'Who decides that the father shall attend his wife's confinement?' The answer is simple, unequivocal: the wife. If the expectant mother wants her husband to be present, and *only* if she wants him, may he attend. Certainly it may be necessary to ask him to leave if some operative procedure is required or some untoward event occurs, but if this has been discussed during pregnancy, no difficulty should arise.

THE BABY AFTER BIRTH

The mother gives one further push, her husband sits beside her whispering to her, encouraging her. Her doctor gently and skilfully steers the baby's head through her vulva, so that it is born. Mucus streams from its nose and mouth; its mouth moves in sucking motions; and it may open its eyes. A further contraction occurs, the mother gently pushes and the baby slips out, still guided by the doctor, to lie on the bed between the mother's legs. It is born. It blinks its eyes; it jerks its arms and legs, clasping and extending its fingers. The umbilical cord, which has been its lifeline for so long, still beats. The nurse sucks its mouth clear of mucus with a rubber tube attached to a suction bulb. The baby takes in a convulsive gasp, and cries for all to hear.

The baby, which has grown from a single cell only visible under the microscope, has now developed into a living being made up of millions upon millions of cells. Some are formed into complex organs; some into bone; some into skin; some into the blood which carries the life-giving oxygen around the body. Its colour becomes pinker and pinker; the umbilical cord stops beating. It is cut. The baby is an independent, perverse, beautiful, irritating, intelligent, dependent, stupid, helpful individual. Which characteristics it will develop depends to a large extent upon its inheritance, but to no small extent upon the upbringing it will receive from its mother and father. The attitudes it will adopt will largely be theirs.

What does it look like, this newborn infant, as it lies crying between its mother's legs, or cuddled within her arms? It will be about 50 cm., or 20 in., long and will weigh anything from 2,500 gm. ($5\frac{1}{2}$ lb.) to 4,500 gm. (10 lb.) – with an average of 3,300 gm. (7 lb. 4 oz.). Its birthweight depends on several factors, such as the physique of its parents, its race, whether or not its mother was ill in pregnancy, and the socio-economic level of its parents. But between these weights, the baby will be normal and healthy, and cause no anxiety.

Its head is rounded, the bones firm, although still separated to leave a diamond-shaped soft space above the forehead and a Y-shaped edge at the back of the head. The baby's brain will grow in the first years of life, and the separation of the bones enables the skull to expand easily. Its head is likely to be covered with fine hair, but some babies are almost bald. You cannot tell from this how its hair will grow later, nor whether it will be prematurely bald! Its ears stand out firmly. Its nose is developed. Its eyes open and blink, but are a slate-grey colour. The real colour of its eyes comes later. Its mouth moves as it makes sucking noises or cries. Its body is rounded; its skin smooth. The lanugo hair which covered it in the uterus has gone, except on its shoulders. Its arms and legs are normal, and the fingers and toes have nails which project beyond their tips. It moves its arms and legs, and if a loud sound is made near it, jerks them convulsively. Its genitals are normal. If a boy, the penis hangs limply, the foreskin projecting beyond its tip, and the testicles are in the scrotum. If a girl, the labia majora are well developed and in contact, so that the vulva is concealed.

It lies peacefully, breathing gently, moving its limbs from time to time. It is this miracle of life which the mother has fed in her womb for the 40 weeks, and has now expelled during the hours of labour (Fig. **14/1**).

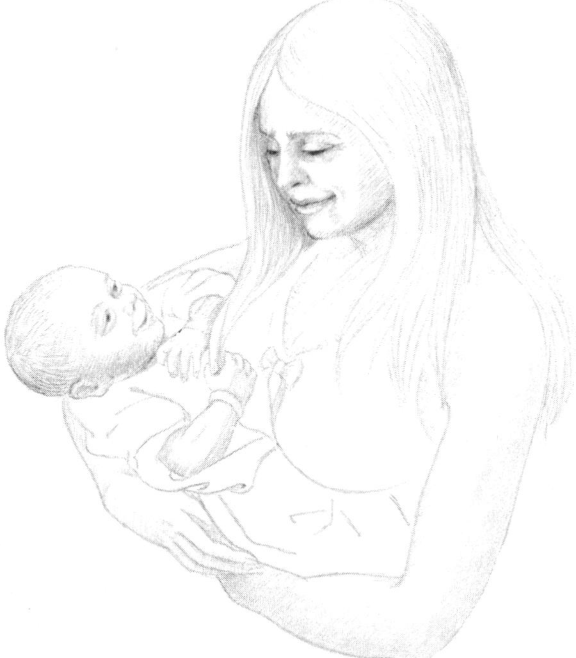

FIG. 14/1. The new-born baby held in its mother's arms

EXAMINATION OF THE BABY

Over 97 per cent of newborn babies are perfect, but in the remaining 3 per cent a defect may be found. The majority of the defects can be treated successfully, often by surgery, provided that they are detected in the first days of life. The doctor will examine the baby systematically and carefully, once its breathing is established. He will examine its head, and look into its mouth to make sure that it has no cleft palate. Because of the pressure on the head of the baby during its passage along the birth-canal, the scalp is often swollen and misshapen, particularly over its posterior part. The swelling is due to congestion of the skin and seeping of fluid into the scalp tissues. It is called a 'caput', and disappears completely within three days. The doctor will then test the movement of the baby's arms and legs, and will pay special attention to its hips, as there is a congenital condition which causes dislocation of the hips. If this is detected and treated by special splinting in the first three months of life, it is completely curable. He will listen to its chest, and examine its abdomen. In particular, he will look at its genitals to make sure that its testicles are normal if it is a boy, and that its vagina is properly formed if it is a girl. Some of the congenital defects cannot be detected by examination – one of these is a strange, and rare, defect called phenylketonuria. If this is not detected early in life, accumulation of a certain substance in the body can lead to mental retardation of the child. Only 1 in 10,000 babies has the defect, but it is now considered that all babies should be tested in the first week of life. The test is quite simple. A sample of the baby's urine is placed on a specially treated piece of paper, which stains if the baby has the defect. Treatment is to give a diet which does not contain phenylalanine, the offending substance.

THE FIRST BATH

It was traditional that soon after birth the baby was weighed (everyone wants to know its weight!) and then bathed. The white, greasy vernix was washed off with soap and water, and the baby powdered and dressed, to be admired by all. It is now known that this method of bathing the baby removed all the protective grease from its skin, and permitted the germs in the air, or blown from its mother's mouth and nose, to settle on the skin, to grow and cause infections. Today, in general, babies are not bathed. Their skin is cleaned with a cleansing agent which is also antiseptic, called pHisohex, but not all the vernix is removed, a fine, invisible layer remaining. Since hospitals have used this method, the incidence of skin infection in babies has dropped very considerably.

CIRCUMCISION

The Jews circumcise their boys on the 8th day of life to fulfil Abram's covenant with God; the Muslims circumcise their boys at puberty as a symbol of reaching manhood; Aboriginal tribes in the Australian desert circumcise their boys, partly ceremonially as an initiation to manhood, partly for hygiene as the desert sand can irritate the foreskin. Circumcision of males has a long religious tradition; but in modern times, in the U.S.A. and Australia particularly, it has become a routine performance, not for religious reasons, but because it is the custom. It is said that mothers demand it, doctors profit by it, and babies cannot complain about it. The reasons given are that removal of the foreskin makes the penis cleaner, prevents masturbation, makes it less sensitive so that ejaculation is delayed in coitus, prevents cancer of the cervix in women, and prevents cancer of the penis in men. The evidence for all these arguments, except the last, is very shaky. The normal foreskin is adherent to the glans of the penis until the infant is a year old. After this time, it can be drawn back, and if the boy is taught to do this, he can keep his foreskin clean. It will not fix his mind on sex. Nor does the absence of a foreskin prevent masturbation, which anyhow is a normal activity. Circumcision does not improve a man's sexual performance, nor does it decrease it: it has no effect. There is no evidence, at all, that secretions which may be found under the foreskin cause cancer of the cervix in women, although many researchers have tried to prove this. The only men who develop cancer of the foreskin are those who are unhygienic. If as children they had been taught to draw back the foreskin and to clean it, cancer would not have occurred.

None of the so-called medical reasons for circumcision is valid, and there is strong evidence that the foreskin *protects* the glans of the penis, which is a delicate, sensitive structure. Circumcised babies may develop tiny ulcers around the 'eye' of the glans, and in a few cases have developed a tightness of the opening, which causes pain on urination. Although these are minor happenings, they suggest that the foreskin has a protective function, especially in infancy.

The decision whether the baby shall be circumcised is, of course, that of the parents, but they should consider the evidence before they decide, and not decide just because 'everyone has it done, and he will feel different from his friends if he hasn't been circumcised'. That is not a reason at all.

CHAPTER 15

Lying-in and going home

The puerperium is the time during which the genital organs, particularly the uterus, slowly return to their non-pregnant state, and when all the other changes which occurred in pregnancy disappear. This period lasts about 8 weeks.

Traditionally the first part of the puerperium was a time of 'lying-in'. It was a time when the woman was kept away from others (particularly men) because she was losing a bloody substance from her vagina and was therefore 'unclean'. It was not realized at that time that the bloody substance, called lochia, was a mixture of blood and the break-down products of tissues discharged as the uterus slowly became smaller and more like a non-pregnant uterus. The tradition of segregation during the lying-in period has largely gone, but many of the surrounding influences, such as the belief that the woman was unclean, have persisted until quite recently.

Up to the last decade, women in the first weeks of the puerperium have been treated as ignorant, idle, ill women who required careful discipline so that they did not damage themselves, and who were expected to fit into hospital routine, however ridiculous, with humbleness and without question. The medical staff 'knew' that if the patient got up before the seventh day after childbirth, prolapse of the uterus would result. So the patient was confined to bed, she found difficulty in passing urine and became constipated. When she did get out of bed, her muscles were so weak that her first steps were faltering. These changes confirmed in the medical attendants' eyes that a puerperal woman was a 'sick woman'. They knew this despite the evidence that in many lands women started work very soon after childbirth without ill effect. Women are often emotional after childbirth which is, after all, a most moving experience, and the mood changes again confirmed the opinion that the patient was ill. For three decades, the baby was separated from the mother and placed in a nursery to be observed by the father like watching fish in an aquarium, and to be brought out to the mother for feeding, who was treated like a battery hen.

Today a new and more sensible approach dominates the care of the puerperal woman. This new philosophy recognizes that the puerperal woman is an intelligent, healthy individual, who has just achieved a most memorable event: she has given birth to a live, healthy baby. She is a person who is subject to emotional moods, for childbirth is a heady thing. She will have to adjust to the demands which the infant will make of her life. This can be difficult, but is less so if she is treated with helpful understanding in the early days of the puerperium, and has received adequate instruction in the 'right approach to parentcraft' during pregnancy.

She is a person who is anxious to see, to touch and to care for her child with the helpful co-operation of the nursing staff. Of course, there may be problems, but most of these can be readily overcome.

The new approach to the puerperium makes three main points. Firstly, although more rest is needed in the early days, the patient should be able to get up and walk about as soon as she wishes. Secondly, in general it is far better from many points of view for the baby to 'room-in' with the mother. Thirdly, mother and baby can go home not on a fixed day, but when conditions are most suitable for them.

Rest

Immediately after the drama of delivery and the excitement of receiving her husband's congratulations, the patient is full of emotional well-being and rather tired. Most women sleep for a while, a few asking for a sedative as they are too excited to sleep. When the mother wakes, she will certainly want to see and hold her baby, and from this time it may well join her in her room. She can get out of bed when she likes, but many women prefer to stay in bed for the first 24 hours, and luxuriate in rest! After this time she should get up, and walk about. It improves the tone of her muscles, it increases the blood flow through her tissues, and it enhances the drainage of the lochia. Moreover, women who practise early ambulation feel much fitter. Swabbing rounds and bed-pans (which are revolting but necessary things) are no longer required. The new mother still requires rest, but she can get this by having a siesta of two hours between lunch-time and visiting time. In many hospitals visiting hours are becoming much more generous, and children are allowed to visit their mother and newly born brother or sister.

Rooming-in

This term implies that for all, or most of the day, the child remains in its cot beside the mother's bed. Of course, if either the mother or child are not fit, perhaps after an operation or because the baby is premature, rooming-in cannot be practised. But most mothers prefer to have the baby with them, instead of seeing it through the nursery window, and touching it only at feeding time. Rooming-in enables the mother to become adjusted to the child, to become accustomed to its behaviour, and to interpret its needs at a time when experienced help is available to reassure her. Rooming-in has the additional advantage that by treating mother and child as a single 'set' or 'unit', cross-infection between babies, always a bug-bear in maternity hospitals, is reduced to a minimum. 'Rooming-in' also seems to make breast-feeding easier. This is so important a subject that it deserves, and gets, a chapter to itself (see Chapter 18).

Going home

The day of discharge should vary to suit the particular mother and her baby. If the mother is normal, as is likely, she should be able to go home whenever she feels fit (once lactation is established), confident that she can cope with the baby. During her stay in hospital, she will have learned to bath the baby, and will have acquired the confidence that it is not as fragile as she had thought. She will have learned to interpret its cry, and to know which cry means 'I'm wet, change me', which 'I'm hungry, feed me,' and which 'I'm full of wind, burp me'! She will have learned how much the baby depends on her, and yet how much it has its own character.

It is wise to remember that babies feel atmosphere. Quite often the change from the noisy hospital to the quiet home is noticed but not understood by the baby. Because of this, in the first two days at home it is irritable and fractious. The mother may think that her milk 'isn't doing it any good', but this is not the reason, and is no occasion for changing to a formula milk. What the baby wants is to feel secure. This it does when it is held close to its mother and cuddled. The prescription for fractious babies in the first few days at home is frequent cuddling.

THE LOCHIA

The three most obvious indications that the mother is no longer expectant are that her stomach is at last flat, or at least flatter than it was, that she has a baby to feed and care for, and that she is discharging lochia. The lochia is the bloody discharge from the uterus which is now shrinking back (or involuting) to its normal size. During pregnancy the uterus was the capsule within which the fetus lived and grew. It protected the fetus from the outside environment; it provided for its nourishment through the placenta; and, finally, by its muscular contractions it expelled the baby into the world. Now these functions are over, the uterus undergoes involution. Immediately after birth it weighs 1,000 gm. ($2\frac{1}{5}$ lb.) and can be felt as a firm, globular bulge reaching up to the umbilicus. By the 14th day after childbirth, it will have shrunk to 350 g. (11 oz.), and can no longer be felt in the abdomen. By the 60th day (8 weeks) after childbirth, it is back to normal size. Involution is brought about by a shrivelling-up of the muscle fibres and the absorption of their substance, partly into the blood stream and partly into the lochia. The lochia is made up of blood from the site where the placenta was attached, and the crumbling of the lining of the uterus which had developed so greatly in pregnancy. In the first 5 days after childbirth, the lochia mostly consists of blood, and is consequently red in colour. For the next 5 to 10 days, it is reddish-brown as the blood loss lessens and more of the uterine lining is expelled. By the 12th day, it has become pale, either yellowish or white; and the discharge persists, varying in amount, for up to six weeks. However, in most cases the discharge has ceased by the end of the third week. The duration of the red lochia varies very considerably, and occasionally it continues for 10 or more days, or episodes of red lochia may recur in the following weeks. They often follow urination, particularly when the patient is not breast-feeding her baby. If the red lochia persists for longer than three weeks, if it becomes as profuse as the amount lost on the first day of a menstrual period, or if clots are passed, the doctor should be consulted.

AFTER-PAINS

After delivery, the uterus does not stop contracting. The contractions continue painlessly for the most part, but in some women, particularly multigravidae, painful contractions persist in the first few days of the puerperium, and may require analgesics. They are especially likely to occur during breast-feeding.

BOWELS

In the past constipation was a problem, but today with early ambulation it is less so. Should a patient become constipated and feel uncomfortable, she should ask for treatment. Usually a gentle laxative, such as Senokot, or a rectal suppository, such as bisacodyl, is given.

URINATION

In the first 24 hours after childbirth, the mother sometimes finds it difficult to pass urine because of the stretching during delivery of the vaginal tissues and the tissues around the bladder. Early ambulation helps, and in fact most women have no trouble.

DIET

The old music hall song 'A little bit of what you fancy does you good' applies in the puerperium. Most women want a meal, certainly a cup of tea, after delivery; and in the puerperium a good wholesome diet, rich in protein and vitamins, with not too much carbohydrate, is needed. Most nutritionists recommend that the puerperal woman who breast-feeds should get at least 2,500 calories a day. The diet of a puerperal mother should be as generous as that she took during pregnancy, with an additional pint of milk a day (some of which may be used in cooking).

ABDOMINAL BINDERS

Formerly it was believed that an abdominal binder was necessary to prevent prolapse and to help the uterus to involute. It is now known that a binder neither prevents a prolapse nor encourages involution, and is not necessary on medical grounds, although a girdle may be required. Some multigravidae feel that the uterus 'flops about', and are more confident and comfortable if they wear a girdle. The choice should be that of the patient, but she should know that the reason for her choice is not medical but psychological.

THIRD DAY BLUES

On about the third day of the puerperium, the excitement of the new baby has diminished a bit. The mother has found that she has an independent, demanding infant to cope with, milk may be filling her breasts which may be tender, and the emotional sensitivity noted earlier may produce a reaction. Depression, mood changes or fits of crying occur for no reason. Everything is going well, but suddenly the patient bursts into a sobbing fit, and after the episode feels better. She knows that she is being silly, but can do nothing to stop it. The thing to remember is that 'third day blues' (which may occur on the fourth or fifth day) are not uncommon, and need sympathetic understanding from the husband and the medical attendants.

EXERCISES

With early ambulation and an intelligent mother, the routine exercises recommended in the past are probably unnecessary. However, many doctors still believe in exercises, and some women require them. Each woman must make up her own mind. The exercises shown in the following diagrams have been used with success in The Women's Hospital (Crown Street), Sydney (Fig. **15/1**).

Exercise 1
To tighten abdominal muscles
Lying on back, one pillow under head. Knees raised up. Place hands on tummy, tighten muscles, relax, and repeat five times. Make sure this is done correctly, the movement is inward. If your chest moves during the exercise the movement is incorrect

Exercise 2
To close separated abdominal muscles
Both hands on tummy, one hand placed over the other, hold the muscles down and against the resistance of your hands, lift head and shoulders off pillow, trying to rise to a sitting position. Repeat five times

1.

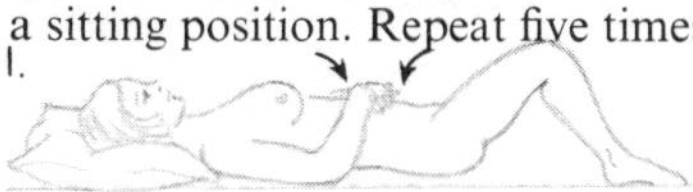

Exercise 3
To tighten the pelvic floor
Press the hollow of the back into the mattress, pull tummy muscles inward, tighten up inside as though preventing the bladder from working

2.

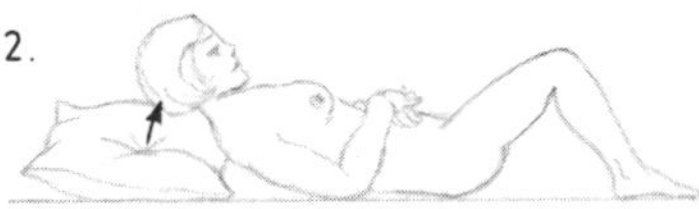

Exercise 4
To restore your waistline
Place hands on waist and tighten as though fastening a very tight skirt. Relax, and repeat five times

3.

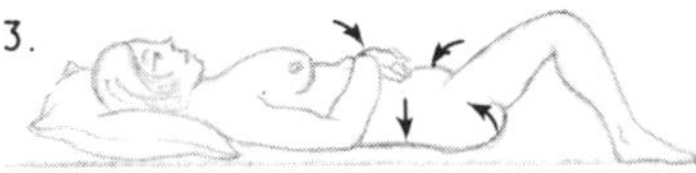

4.

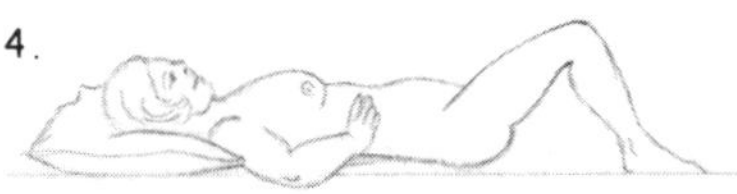

Exercise 5
For circulation and leg strengthening
Lying on back with legs straight.
(a) Move feet up and down
(b) Move feet round in circles
(c) Feet straight up, toes curled over
(d) Tighten the kneecap and tense leg muscles
(e) Ankles crossed, press thighs together, tighten up inside

5.

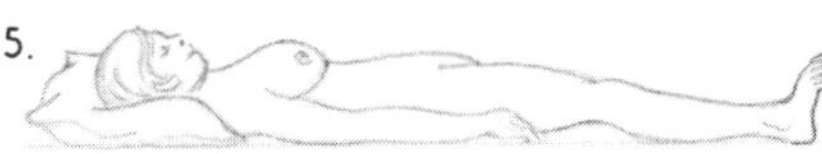

6a.

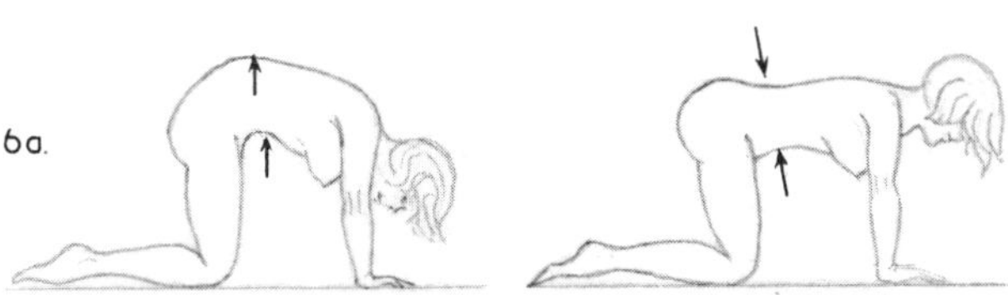

Exercise 6
Kneeling
(a) Kneeling on hands and knees, first arch and then hollow the back, keep tummy muscles tight.
(b) Then move head and hip to the right. Relax and then move head and hip to the left

6b.

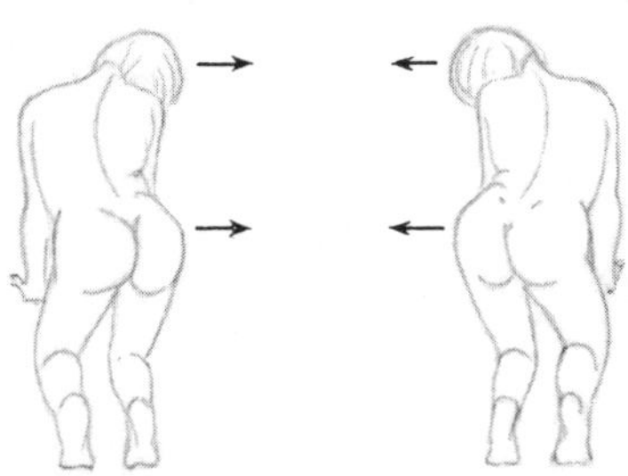

FIG. 15/1. Postnatal exercises. These exercises are to restore your muscle tone, and your figure after childbirth. The exercises should be done daily, each one at least five times, for a period of three months

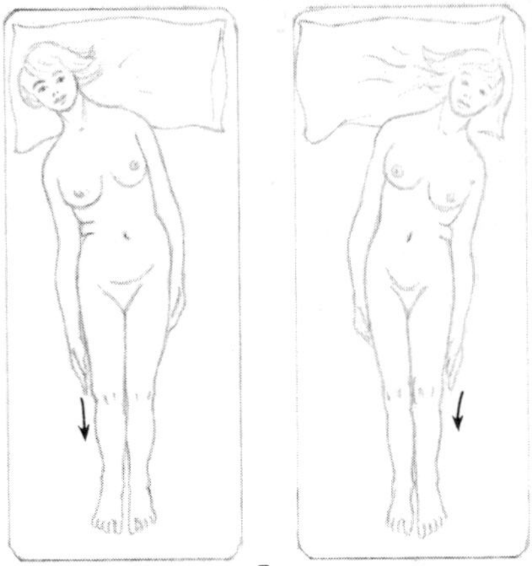
7a.

Exercise 7
Stretching exercises
Lying on back
(a) Tummy muscles tighten, stretch arms down to each side alternately as though trying to grasp ankles. Relax, and repeat five times
Lying on side
(b) Lying on the left side, tighten tummy muscles, stretch top arm and top leg down so that body is in one long line. Relax, and repeat the same exercise lying on the right side. Relax, and repeat five times

7b.
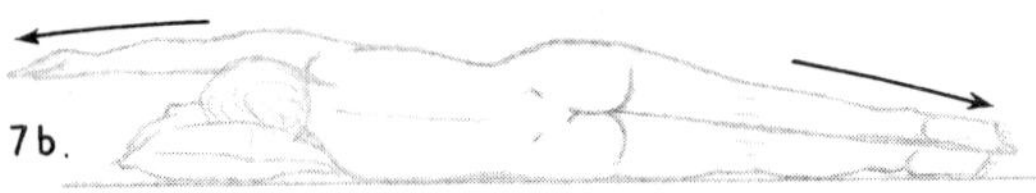

8.
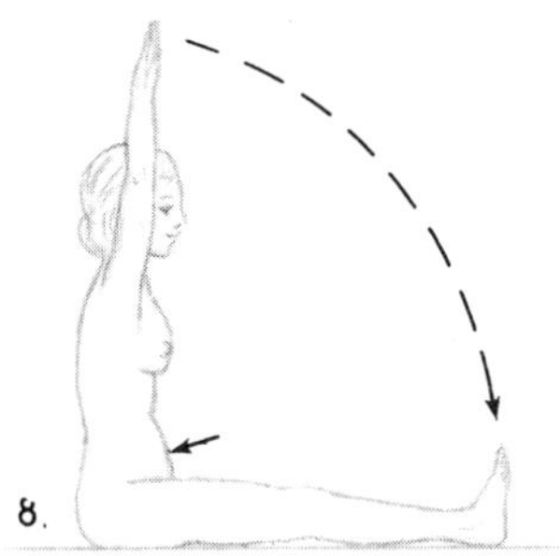

9.
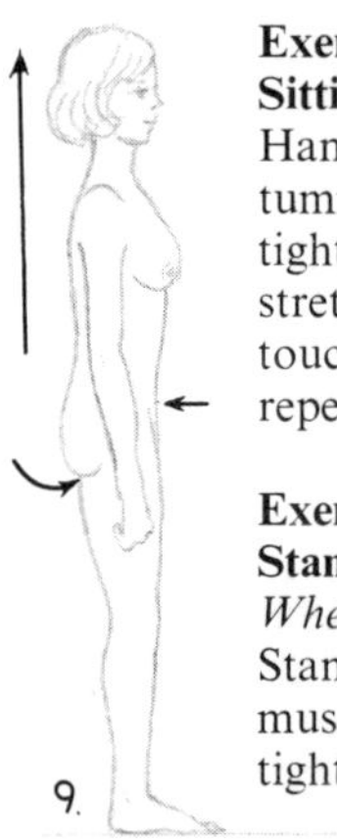

Exercise 8
Sitting up
Hands above head, tummy muscles tightened, tighten internally, stretch forward and touch toes. Relax, and repeat five times

Exercise 9
Standing
When allowed to stand
Stand tall, tummy muscles pulled inward, tighten up inside

10.
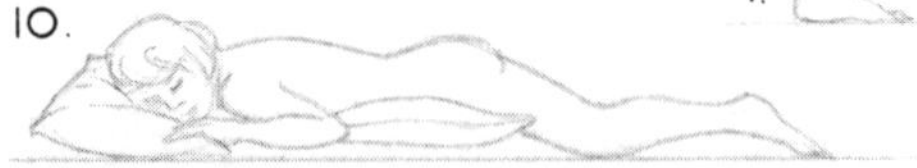

Exercise 10
Lying face down
Spend at least 20 minutes lying face down, one pillow under the face, one pillow under the tummy, tightening the muscles

1.

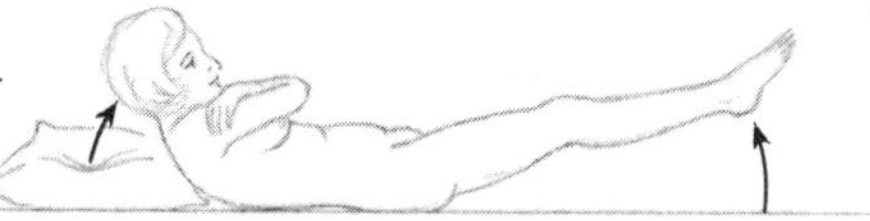

Exercise 1
Lying on back on bed, abdominal muscles tightened, arms folded across chest, raise head and shoulders and legs slowly. Slowly lower

2.

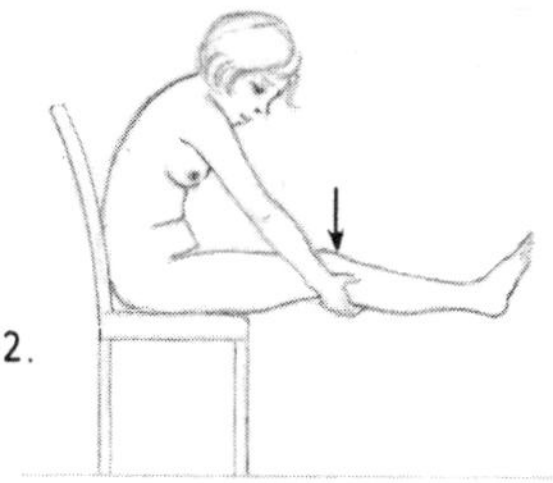

Exercise 2
Sitting on chair, legs extended, abdominal muscles tightened, place hands below knees and press legs down into the hands. Hold this position to the count of six

3.

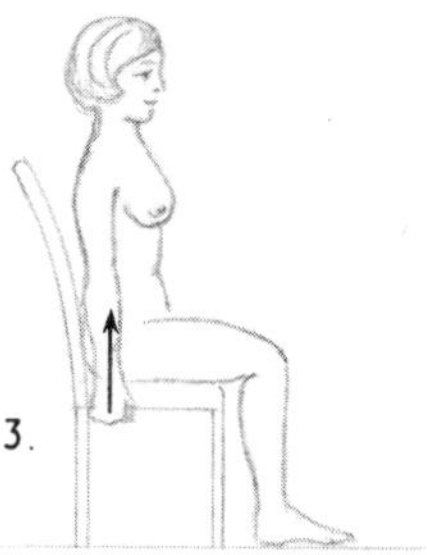

Exercise 3
Sitting on chair, place hands under the seat of the chair, feet firmly on floor and tighten all muscles. Imagine lifting self and chair towards the ceiling. Hold to count of six

4.

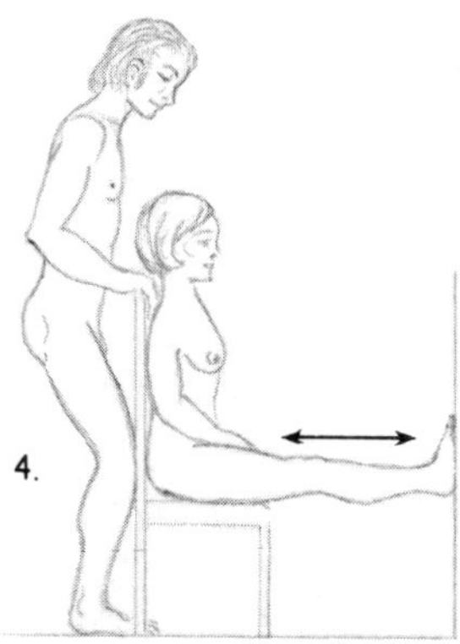

Exercise 4
Sitting on chair, feet on wall, push away from wall with abdominal muscles braced

FIG. 15/1 (continued). Advanced postnatal exercises. These exercises require greater muscular energy, two are 'isometric', and all can be done when you feel ready

VISITORS

In the matter of visitors, attitudes are changing. At one stage only the husband might visit, and this had a venerable tradition. In the seventeenth century, a great French obstetrician referring to the habit of holding a party on the third day of the puerperium when the child was baptised, wrote, 'Though there is scarce any of the company, which do not drink her health, yet by the noise they make in her ears, she loses it'.

Today it is realized that this attitude is unnecessarily restrictive. The husband should be allowed to visit at any time of the day, and it is nonsense to say that this interferes with hospital routine; the hospital is there for the patient, and not the patient for the hospital. Other visitors should be permitted at specific times each day, but should inquire first if they may visit. Each woman feels differently about visitors: some women want very few, preferring to be with their husbands; others want to keep in touch with their friends. But the friends should realize that the demands of a young baby, and the odd schedule of early waking found in hospitals, may make the mother very tired. For this reason, visits should be cut short. The visitor can always see the mother when she goes home, and nowadays this is tending to be sooner after childbirth.

THE POSTNATAL CHECK-UP

It is usual for the doctor to request that the puerperal mother return to see him between 6 and 8 weeks after confinement. This postnatal check-up is of considerable importance, as it enables the doctor to make sure that all is well, and it gives the mother the opportunity to discuss any problems which may still cause her anxiety. Many doctors want to see the baby as well as the mother.

The examination is quite painless, and the extent of the investigations which need to be made depends on whether the pregnancy and labour were normal or complicated. If they were normal, the doctor will merely palpate the mother's abdomen, examine the cervix with a speculum, and perhaps take a further 'Pap smear'. He will also do a pelvic examination so that he can determine if the uterus has involuted properly. If the mother has any complaints, he will deal with these.

In recent years, the postnatal visit has provided the opportunity to discuss with the doctor the subjects of birth control for herself and immunization programmes for her baby. These two matters are today probably the most important aspects of the postnatal visit.

SEXUAL INTERCOURSE AFTER CHILDBIRTH

Although it is usual to await the postnatal examination before sexual intercourse is resumed, this is not strictly necessary. Provided that coitus does not cause pain, it may be resumed once the lochia has ceased. Whether or not sexual intercourse is resumed is a matter for the couple to decide, the wife making the final decision.

THE RETURN OF MENSTRUATION AFTER CHILDBIRTH

If the mother is breast-feeding, menstruation does not usually return for about 24 weeks, or 6 months. Ten per cent of women menstruate by 10 weeks after childbirth, 20 per cent by 20 weeks, and 60 per cent by 30 weeks. Ovulation is unusual before the 20th week after childbirth, but about 2 per cent of lactating women do ovulate before this time. However, pregnancy rarely occurs in the first 20 weeks of the puerperium. Even if the menstrual periods start, breast-feeding can be continued as the quality of the milk is not altered during menstruation.

In modern Western society, about 70 per cent of mothers do not breast-feed. These women are at much greater risk of pregnancy, as in over 80 per cent menstruation and ovulation have begun by the 10th week after the birth of the child.

CHAPTER 16

The Rhesus factor and other matters

THE RHESUS PROBLEM

Until 1940 the reason why a number of babies were born dead, swollen with fluid and looking like small Buddhas, puzzled many obstetricians. They were also puzzled by the fact that some babies, who were apparently normal at birth, became severely jaundiced and died within a few days. The explanation of these two phenomena suddenly became clear. In 1940 two scientists had noted that the red blood cells of certain women had a strange substance, called an antigen, attached to their surface. If these red blood cells were injected, as in a blood transfusion, into the blood stream of another person, they would provoke the formation of substances called antibodies in that person's blood stream. But this reaction only occurred if the person receiving the blood transfusion did not have any red cells of her own which had antigen on their surface. If she had such cells, no reaction occurred.

Once the antibodies were formed, they attached themselves to the antigen sites on the injected, or foreign, red blood cells; and, in a complicated way clumped (or agglutinated) them. The red blood cells agglutinated in this way first became swollen, then burst and were destroyed. (In a way, this is similar to what happens when a heart is transplanted into another person, and is then 'rejected' by that person.) During their experiments with the antigen, the doctors had prepared a serum by injecting the red cells of Rhesus monkeys into guinea pigs, and had found that all Rhesus monkeys had the antigen attached to their red blood cells. Because of this, they called the antigen the Rhesus antigen, or the Rhesus factor. They then decided to study how many Americans had the Rhesus factor attached to their red blood cells. After much investigation, they found that 85 per cent of Americans had the Rhesus factor attached to their red blood cells, and 15 per cent had no Rhesus factor on their red blood cells. Those with the factor they called Rhesus positive; those without it Rhesus negative. Further investigations of other races showed some differences. For example, Europeans had the same proportion of Rhesus negative people; but in North India, the incidence of Rhesus negative people was only 10 per cent; and in South India less than 5 per cent; whilst Rhesus negative people were almost never found amongst Chinese. This strange difference of numbers of Rhesus negative people in different races is not understood.

More importantly from the point of view of our discussion, other investigators remembered the unexplained deaths of the jaundiced babies, and inquired what was the Rhesus group of their mothers. In every case the mother had been Rhesus negative and the father had been Rhesus positive. And in every case the mother had previously received a blood transfusion, or had one or more previous pregnancies.

A woman marries a man not because of his blood group, but because he is attractive to her, or has qualities which appeal to her. In short, because she is in love with him. Since 85 per cent of people are Rhesus positive and 15 per cent Rhesus negative, the odds are that in 10 per cent of marriages the wife may be Rhesus negative and the husband Rhesus positive. At some stage, quite naturally, they decide to have a baby. Because it inherits half of its genes from its father, it may be Rhesus positive or it may be Rhesus negative. If it is Rhesus negative, no problem arises; but if it is Rhesus positive, problems may occur with a later pregnancy, although the first baby will not be affected. During the pregnancy, the Rhesus positive baby grows happily in its mother's womb, but off and on in late pregnancy tiny numbers of its Rhesus positive red blood cells may seep across the placenta and enter the mother's blood stream, where they are destroyed. At delivery, however, much larger amounts of fetal blood get into the mother's blood stream. The amount may be too great to be destroyed immediately, and the surviving cells are recognized as being foreign invaders, which have Rhesus positive badges on them! The mother's defence system goes into action and special commando cells, called immuno-competent cells, manufacture the destroying substance (or antibody) which attaches itself to the foreign Rhesus positive cells, coats their surface, clumps them and literally blows them apart.

The mother's defence system, once stimulated, remains ever on the alert should any further Rhesus positive cells enter her body.

The couple decide to have a further child. Again it inherits half its genes from its father, and again it may be Rhesus positive. If it is, a strange thing now happens. The anti-Rh antibody which the mother's immuno-competent cells have continued to manufacture circulates through her blood stream, and because of its peculiar shape is able to pass through the placenta and enter the blood stream of the fetus. This does not happen in very early pregnancy, but becomes more and more likely as pregnancy advances. In the blood stream it meets the baby's normal Rhesus positive red blood cells, and coats them so that they burst. The burst red cells release a substance called bilirubin, which accumulates in the baby's blood and some of it is excreted into the amniotic sac in the baby's urine. As its red blood cells are destroyed, the baby becomes progressively more anaemic. If too many red blood cells are destroyed, it becomes so anaemic that it is bloated, Buddha-like and dies. If fewer red blood cells are destroyed, the baby remains alive but is born anaemic and jaundiced from the accumulation of bilirubin in its blood.

Once these facts had been discovered, it was possible to find out firstly if the Rhesus negative mother had been stimulated to manufacture antibodies, by doing a test on her blood; and secondly, to determine how badly the baby was likely to be affected, by taking a sample of the amniotic fluid and estimating the amount of bilirubin in it. This test on the amniotic fluid was done first at about 28 weeks, and repeated once or twice more. The object of all these tests was to find out when it was more dangerous for the baby to be inside the uterus than to be born. Once born, its damaged blood could be replaced in an 'exchange transfusion' by Rhesus negative blood, which the antibodies could not attack since the red cells had no antigen on their suface. The transfused blood kept the baby alive whilst such antibodies as remained slowly decayed over the following weeks. Some babies needed further 'topping-up' transfusions, but by six weeks of life, they were all well. None of the antibodies the mother had transferred to them remained, and their Rhesus problem was over. Using these methods of care, most Rhesus affected babies now survive, but a few still die in the uterus. A New Zealand doctor thought that some of these could be saved if they could be given a transfusion whilst still in the womb, to help them survive there until they were slightly more mature and able to survive outside. He suggested that very badly affected babies, who were not yet Buddha-like but were still less than 34 weeks mature, should be treated in this way. It is a complicated procedure to perform an 'intra-uterine transfusion', but one-third of the babies treated in this way survive.

Today a treatment is available which will almost eliminate the problem, at least for those Rhesus negative women who have not started to manufacture antibodies. Scientists in Britain and the U.S.A. have discovered that Rhesus negative women can be protected by giving them an injection of a special antibody, made in the blood of Rhesus negative volunteers. The injection is only useful if given to a Rhesus negative mother who has not yet made any antibodies against Rhesus positive blood. The scientists believe that the special antibody works by coating and destroying any fetal Rhesus positive red blood cells which have entered the mother's blood stream during labour. The injection is painless, and is effective if given up to 72 hours after birth.

Provided the mother has been tested in pregnancy so that it is known whether she is Rhesus negative, and a sample of the cord blood of the baby is tested and found to be Rhesus positive, the special injection can be obtained and injected into the mother. This will protect her completely against the 'Rhesus problem'.

A number of doctors with different skills – immunologists, haematologists, obstetricians and paediatricians – have combined their activities to obtain this result. It is an example of team-work in medicine for the benefit of women.

GERMAN MEASLES (RUBELLA)

The careful observations by Dr. Gregg in Sydney in 1941 first brought to our attention the dangers of German measles in the first half of pregnancy. German measles (rubella) is caused by a virus which can cross the placenta and infect the baby. It is a peculiar virus, as it prefers to grow in tissue which is just forming. Before the 10th week of pregnancy it has a wonderful opportunity, for the heart, the ears, and the skull of the fetus are forming at this time.

If the virus gets into the tissue, the heart may be damaged, the hearing impaired, the eyes may develop cataracts, and the skull may not expand. Because of these serious complications affecting more than half of the babies, many doctors believe that a therapeutic abortion should be performed if a woman develops rubella in the first 12 weeks of pregnancy.

Some pregnant women come into contact with a case of rubella, either in their own family or in a neighbour's. Until very recently it was the custom to give them an injection of 'gamma globulin', which was painful, but which was said to protect the fetus from the virus. It is now known that the injections of 'gamma globulin' are of no value in protecting the babies.

It would be sad if nothing more could be said, but it can. A test has now been developed which will tell if a patient has had rubella, and once you have had rubella, you are protected for all time. A specimen of the person's blood is taken and the test made. In Australia, the U.S.A. and probably in most other countries, it has been found that more than 85 per cent of women have rubella before they reach the age of 16. The other 15 per cent have not had rubella, but a vaccine is available (at present on trial) which will be able to give these women a mild attack of rubella. They will not know that they have had rubella, but they will be protected.

Testing to tell if a woman has had rubella is rather complicated and expensive, and because of this the vaccine is going to be offered to all schoolgirls when they reach the age of 14. But since many women do not know if they have had rubella, it is expected that they will be tested if they wish. The most suitable time for testing to see if a woman has had rubella is when she decides to marry, or just before she decides to have a baby. If her test is positive, she knows that her baby is in no danger of being damaged by the rubella virus. If the test is negative, she can be given an injection of rubella vaccine. If she decides that she will have the injection, she must take precautions to avoid becoming pregnant for two months after the injection. After that time she will have become protected against rubella, and there is no chance of her baby being damaged by the rubella virus.

GENERAL DISEASE AND PREGNANCY

Two conditions, in particular, require extra care during pregnancy. These are diabetes and heart disease. Any woman who is a diabetic or has heart disease should see her doctor as early as possible in pregnancy. The amount of insulin the diabetic requires during pregnancy fluctuates, and proper control of the diabetes can only be obtained by regular blood tests for sugar. In diabetes it is usual for the mother to be admitted to hospital at about the 32nd week, and to be delivered in the 37th week, but each case requires individual attention. Regular antenatal visits at short intervals are essential, and often the patient's doctor will seek the help of a physician who is interested in the disease. In diabetes, the help and co-operation of the expectant mother is essential if she is to have a live baby.

The patient with heart disease usually has no trouble in pregnancy, but in the more severe forms may require to go into hospital at about the 30th week for bed-rest. As is the case in diabetes, regular, frequent visits to her doctor throughout pregnancy are essential. She must also avoid putting on too much weight, which means that she must eat a balanced diet, avoiding excess carbohydrates, sweets and sugar. She must also avoid becoming anaemic, and her doctor will undoubtedly test her blood for anaemia and prescribe iron tablets. She must not omit to take these.

BREECH BABIES

In the middle of pregnancy, because the fetus is small and the amniotic sac relatively large, the baby tends to move around a good deal. At this time about 40 per cent of babies present with their bottom nearest the mother's pelvis. These are called breech presentations. By the 28th week, the percentage has dropped to 15 per cent; by the 34th week to 6 per cent; and by the 40th week less than 4 per cent of babies still present by the breech. The reason is that as pregnancy advances, there is more room for the legs in the upper part of the uterus, and the baby gets into the most comfortable position! Most of the babies which remain as breech presentations have their legs straight, the feet under the chin (Fig. **16/1**).

In the past breech babies often died during delivery, but today with skilled attention, teamwork by the obstetrician, the anaesthetist

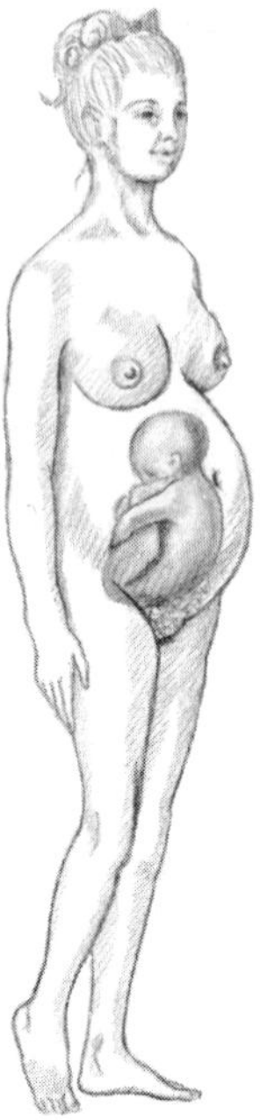

FIG. 16/1. The breech baby

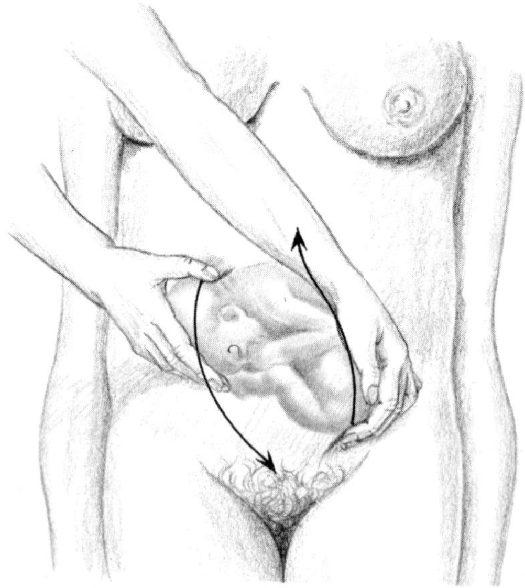

FIG. 16/2. Turning a breech baby

and the nurses, these problems have been overcome. However, if the expectant mother still has a breech presentation when the pregnancy has reached 34 weeks' gestation, the doctor may try to 'turn it'. This is a simple manipulation, and is not painful, so the expectant mother does not need an anaesthetic. He is very gentle as he attempts to do the 'external version', and if the baby does not turn easily, he does not persist (Fig. **16/2**). Before the manipulation, the mother should be sure that her bowels and bladder are empty, and that she is relaxed. If the doctor fails to turn the baby, he will probably ask the mother to have an X-ray to make sure that the pelvic bones and the cavity of the pelvis have a normal shape.

Most breech babies are born easily, after a labour which is no longer or more difficult than if the baby was 'head-down', or more correctly was a cephalic, or vertex, presentation. But in certain cases, particularly if the baby is very large, a Caesarean section will be performed.

The mother whose baby remains as a breech need have no anxiety, and when her baby is born she will see that its head has a beautiful round shape. When the baby lies as a cephalic presentation, its head is often temporarily distorted for a few hours after birth. It is of no consequence to the baby, and the shape becomes normal very rapidly.

MULTIPLE PREGNANCY

It is quite normal for most mammals to have a multiple pregnancy or litter. The human female usually only has a single baby in each pregnancy, but one pregnancy in 90 is a twin pregnancy; one pregnancy in 90 x 90 is a triplet pregnancy; and quadruplets occur once in 90 x 90 x 90 pregnancies. There are two ways in which a multiple pregnancy can occur: either two (or more) eggs are released from the ovary at one time, and are fertilized by two different spermatozoa; or the single fertilized egg cell may completely divide at the stage of the blastocyst, and then *two* individuals develop, but have a single placenta. The first kind of twins are fraternal twins, who are no closer to each other in characteristics than any brother and sister. The second kind are identical twins, and are mirror images of each other. The fraternal twins make up 75 per cent of all twin pregnancies; identical twins only 25 per cent.

Twins are more frequent in African and Asian countries, and this is due to the higher proportion of fraternal twins, as identical twins occur equally often whatever the race or age of the mother. Amongst Caucasians, or Europeans, fraternal twins occur more frequently in families with a history of twins, in older women, amongst women who have had several children previously, and after injection of drugs which induce ovulation.

Each twin is always lighter than a singleton baby at the same stage of pregnancy, although, of course, the combined weight of the twins is greater than that of the singleton. Because of this, twins tend to be underweight at birth. As well, the size of the twins can vary very considerably. The difference between them is greater when they are identical twins, as one of them is greedy and takes the greater part of the nourishment which arrives through the placenta. Inside the womb, the twins lie side by side. In late pregnancy, it has been shown that in 45 per cent of cases both lie with the head over the mother's pelvis; in 25 per cent the leading twin has its head down, and the other twin is a breech; in 10 per cent the breech leads the head; and in 10 per cent both are breeches (Fig. **16/3**).

The doctor may suspect twins when he finds that the uterus is larger than he anticipated calculating from the date of the last period (see Fig. **8/3**). There are other causes for the undue enlargement of the womb, but twins is the most common cause. It is possible he will be able to feel both babies, but this is unusual before the 28th week of pregnancy, by which time the expectant mother may herself suspect that she has twins. If the doctor is uncertain, he will arrange for an X-ray picture, which will show the two babies and their positions in the uterus. X-rays are usually avoided before the 24th week of pregnancy to reduce the risk of radiation to the babies.

A multiple pregnancy is a little more risky than a single pregnancy, but provided the expectant mother attends regularly for antenatal care, the risk is small. 'Toxaemia of pregnancy' occurs more frequently, as does anaemia. Many doctors prevent anaemia by giving the expectant mother iron tablets with a tiny amount of folic acid added, from about the 30th week of pregnancy. In late pregnancy, twins usually impose more discomfort on the expectant mother, than does a single infant. Her abdomen feels heavier, she has more backache, and swelling of her ankles and legs is quite common. It has also been found that twin pregnancies tend to end prematurely,

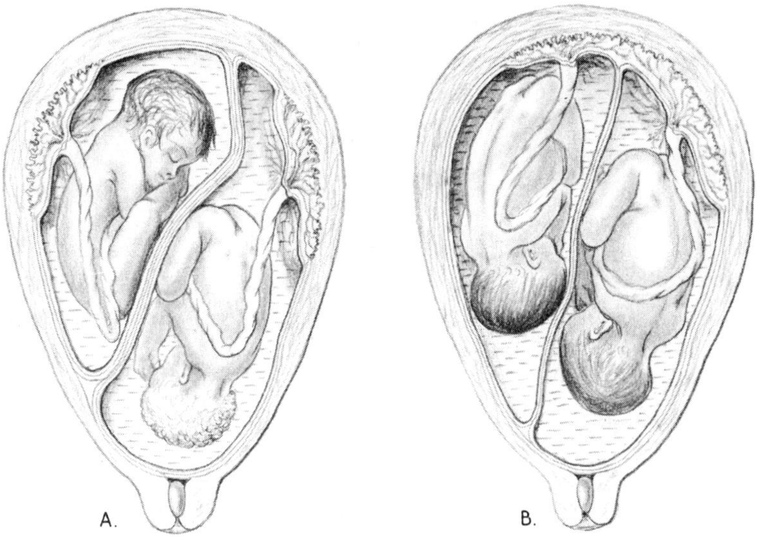

FIG. 16/3. Twins
(a) Fraternal twins from the chance fertilization of two ova.
(b) Identical twins, from the fertilization of a single ovum and its later division into two identical embryos.

and about one-quarter of twin babies are delivered by the 36th week. This premature rate can be reduced considerably with good antenatal care, and if the mother rests for a good deal of the day from the 32nd week on. She should certainly give up work, if she can afford to, by the 28th week.

Contrary to popular belief, labour in a twin pregnancy is no longer than in a single pregnancy, but the delivery of one or both of the twins is often aided by the doctor. There is often an interval of about 10 minutes between the birth of the twins, but no doctor today would allow an interval as long as the 65 days which was reported some years ago.

Finally, an old myth should be demolished. Twins are not less fertile than singletons when in their turn they marry.

AGE AND OBSTETRIC PERFORMANCE

Examination of the records from very large numbers of pregnancies in many countries has been made to see if age has any effect, good or otherwise, on obstetric performance. There has been surprising agreement that the least complications in pregnancy and during childbirth are found if the mother has been well-nourished from childhood, has some knowledge of what happens in pregnancy, is more than 61 inches tall, not over-weight nor emaciated, and aged between 18 and 25! Of course, this does not mean that younger or old mothers, fat or excessively thin mothers, or short women do not perform well. They do, but there is apparently a greater chance that complications may arise.

The teenage mother

There has been concern, particularly in the U.S.A., Britain and Australia, about the increasing number of teenage mothers, particularly those under the age of 17 who are unmarried. In Eastern countries, it is normal for marriage to take place soon after puberty, and for consumation of the marriage to occur either then or, as with Hindus, two to three years later, so that teengage pregnancies are not unusual. There is nothing to suggest that the teenage mother is in any way disadvantaged in pregnancy, provided that she seeks antenatal care as early as possible. In a study of teenage mothers which we have conducted in Sydney, we found that if the girl received antenatal check-ups, she had a slightly greater chance of developing 'toxaemia of pregnancy' than her older sisters, and was a bit more likely to become anaemic. The duration of labour was not increased; in fact labour seemed easier, and the average birth weight of her baby was not different from that of her older sisters, nor was there any increased risk that her baby would be born dead or die soon after birth. If the girl did not attend the antenatal clinic until late in pregnancy, as happened with many of the unmarried teenage mothers, we found that there was twice the chance that she would develop 'toxaemia of pregnancy' or become anaemic; and although the duration and conduct of labour was not altered, she had double the risk of losing her baby.

The importance of these observations is that every teenage girl who becomes pregnant, whether she is married or not, should seek antenatal care as early as possible. She need not be worried that the doctors and nurses will condemn her for getting pregnant–they will not; and they will be happy that she has had the sense to come along so that her pregnancy and labour may be made as easy as possible. Often the unmarried girl has many problems to face, and most maternity hospitals have a staff of qualified social workers who can advise and reassure her, can give her confidence, and talk to her with kindness and wisdom.

The older primigravida

About 5 per cent of women, usually of the higher socio-economic groups, delay becoming pregnant until they are more than 30 years old. Such a patient is called an 'older primigravida', rather than the previous term 'elderly primigravida', which is somewhat insulting to the expectant mother! The older primigravida may develop more complications in pregnancy than her younger sister, and because of this she should obtain antenatal care as early as possible in pregnancy so that any complications can be diagnosed and treated quickly.

The older primigravida has three times the risk of developing 'toxaemia of pregnancy', and a slightly greater chance of having a breech baby or a twin pregnancy than her younger sister. As 'toxaemia' can be controlled by bed-rest and drugs, this is of no great danger provided she is receiving competent antenatal care. Labour in the older primigravida tends to last rather longer than amongst her younger primigravid sisters, and her baby's birth needs to be helped by forceps or Caesarean section more frequently. Even so, only about 10 per cent of these patients require Caesarean section, whilst 35 per cent are delivered by forceps.

The grande multigravida

This term was first used in Dublin to describe those women who have had at least four previous pregnancies. These mothers are more likely to have complications in pregnancy and labour than women who have had fewer children, and the risk is greater if the mother is aged 35 or more. Unfortunately, this is the patient who most frequently neglects to obtain antenatal care. If she does seek antenatal care, the chance of a complication occurring in pregnancy or labour is greatly reduced. She is more likely to develop bleeding in pregnancy, and 'toxaemia of pregnancy' is a little more frequent. Although she may deliver a bigger baby, labour is usually quite rapid. However, she has a risk of bleeding after delivery until action is taken.

These findings emphasize the importance of regular antenatal visits, and delivery in a well-equipped hospital under the care of a well-trained doctor.

CHAPTER 17

Pregnancy complications

In more than 70 per cent of pregnancies the antenatal period and the confinement are completely normal. In the remaining 30 per cent of pregnancies conditions may appear which require treatment so that a live, healthy baby is delivered by a healthy mother. The detection of the conditions whilst they are still mild is one of the purposes of good antenatal care. It is for this reason that the expectant mother was recommended to make regular visits to her doctor as described in Chapter 10. It can safely be said that the conditions only prove serious if the expectant mother fails to attend her doctor at the first sign of abnormality.

What are the signs which should lead an expectant mother to contact her doctor immediately, so that she may visit him or he may visit her at her house?

They can be listed as follows:

1. Bleeding in the first half of pregnancy, with or without cramping abdominal pains.
2. Severe abdominal pains in the first weeks of pregnancy.
3. Bleeding with or without abdominal pain in the second half of pregnancy.
4. Swelling of the fingers or face, particularly if accompanied by headaches and blurring of vision.
5. A gush of water from the vagina in the second half of pregnancy.

BLEEDING IN THE FIRST HALF OF PREGNANCY

The usual cause of bleeding in the first half of pregancy is that the expectant mother is threatening to abort. About one pregnancy in seven ends as a 'spontaneous' abortion, which is the correct term for the lay euphemism of 'miscarriage'. All that the word abortion means is that the embryo or fetus is expelled from the uterus; it does not mean that the expectant mother has gone to an abortionist – that is called an 'induced' or 'criminal' abortion. In at least three-quarters of cases, the reason for a spontaneous abortion is that the fetus was not properly formed, and Nature is getting rid of it. In a few cases an abortion may follow a severe fever, such as pneumonia, and in even fewer cases the doctor may find an abnormality of the uterus or a weakness of the cervix. In the past a retroverted uterus (one which is 'bent back'), excessive coitus, fatigue, 'undue exertion', or a 'severe shock' were blamed for the occurrence of an abortion. It is now known that none of these causes an abortion.

The first sign of an impending, or threatened, abortion is usually bleeding. This may merely be some slight irregular 'spotting' of blood, followed after a few hours or days by a moderate discharge of blood from the vagina, which may resemble a menstrual period.

In other cases the bleeding is heavier at the start, and may be accompanied by some slight cramping pains, resembling period pains. Despite the anxiety caused to the expectant mother by the appearance of these symptoms, it is reassuring that more than 80 per cent of cases of threatened abortion settle down, and the pregnancy continues. If this happens, the baby will certainly be quite normal.

The expectant mother should inform her doctor at once if she bleeds in early pregnancy. He may suggest that she goes to bed for a few days, and that coitus is avoided for a couple of weeks. If she is anxious, as she may well be, he will probably prescribe a sedative to calm her down. The sedative also reduces the sensitivity of the uterus and calms it down. For many years a variety of vitamins and hormones were given to patients with threatened abortion. A favourite was progesterone, or one of the chemical substitutes for the natural drug. A great number of women received expensive injections or took expensive tablets of the progesterone-like drugs. There is now clear, certain evidence that neither progesterone, nor its chemical substitutes, is of any value in the treatment of threatened abortion, apart from a psychological value. There are cheaper and more effective ways of providing the expectant mother with the psychological support, and a wise, honorable New York obstetrician once recommended 'T.L.C. frequently every day'. T.L.C. stands for tender, loving care!

In 20 per cent of cases of threatened abortion, the bleeding increases and abdominal cramps become severe. The abortion is now probably inevitably going to occur. Many women who abort do not notice the threatened and inevitable stages, as they succeed each other too quickly. These patients complain of sudden bleeding and painful cramps, and on going to the toilet, expel 'something' from the vagina. The doctor should be called at once, and everything which has been discharged from the vagina should be kept for his inspection. If this is done, it makes his task much easier. On his arrival, the doctor usually gives the patient a pain-relieving drug, and then performs a pelvic examination. This will tell him if all of the fetus and the placenta have been expelled, or if some remains inside the uterus. If it does, the doctor will certainly wish the patient to go to hospital so that he may 'clean out', or curette, the cavity of the womb.

Statistics show that if a patient has seven pregnancies in her lifetime, one is likely to end as an abortion. The fact that a patient has had an abortion in one pregnancy does not mean that it will happen again. If she has an abortion, there is an 80 per cent chance that the next pregnancy will produce a live, normal, healthy baby; if she has two abortions in succession, the chance of the next pregnancy producing a live, healthy baby is 75 per cent; and even after three abortions, one after the other, she still has a 70 per cent chance of producing a live, healthy baby with her next pregnancy.

In fact, however disappointed an expectant mother may be, she should not be anxious if a pregnancy ends as an abortion; her next pregnancy has every chance of being normal.

Most threatened abortions occur in the first 12 weeks of pregnancy, but a few women complain of vaginal bleeding between the 12th and 28th week of pregnancy. In these cases the cause may be a weakness of the neck of the womb (the cervix), and women with this condition usually have repeated abortions. Not all repeated abortions are due to this condition, however. Normally the cervical canal is quite firm, and does not increase in size although the uterus is enlarging as the fetus grows. In women who have a weakness of the cervix, it begins to open more and more after the 12th week of pregnancy for some reason, and eventually an abortion occurs. The cases are fairly rare, but a live baby can be obtained in three-quarters of them if a stitch is placed around the cervix and then pulled tight, like pulling the string around the mouth of a purse. The operation is very simple, and most successful if the case has been properly selected. In other words, only a very few women have this weakness of the cervix, and the operation is therefore not often needed.

Recurrent, or habitual abortion does require investigation, and if a woman has the misfortune to have three or more abortions in succession, she would be wise to consult her doctor. He will make several investigations, which include a full physical examination and a pelvic examination. As well he usually makes some laboratory tests to make sure that the woman has no undetected disease. and often takes an X-ray picture of the uterus after injecting an oily substance into it.

ABDOMINAL PAIN IN EARLY PREGNANCY

An expectant mother who develops severe abdominal pain, fainting and slight bleeding in early pregnancy should at once consult her doctor, as she may have an ectopic pregnancy. In this condition the fertilized egg plants itself in the lining of the oviduct. This lining is thin, and is surrounded by a thin muscle wall. As the embryo grows, its placenta eats into the muscle wall, which eventually bursts. Ectopic pregnancy is not too common, occurring in 1 in 150 pregnancies. The treatment is surgery to remove the damaged portion of the oviduct. Of course, as every woman has two oviducts, she can become pregnant again after an ectopic pregnancy.

BLEEDING IN THE SECOND HALF OF PREGNANCY

Bleeding from the birth-canal occurs in the second half of pregnancy in about three per cent of women. Usually they are women who have previously delivered children, and primigravidae uncommonly develop this complication. If an expectant mother bleeds sufficiently to soil a sanitary pad, or to make a large stain on her clothes or her bed sheets, she should call her doctor at once. He may visit her in her house, or he may insist that she go into hospital immediately where he will examine her.

Bleeding in the second half of pregnancy is called 'antepartum haemorrhage'. Apart from the few cases due to local conditions of the cervix, there are two main causes, which were first distinguished in 1775 by Dr. Edward Rigby in Norwich. At that time maternity care was conducted by untrained midwives, and they only attended the woman when she was in labour. If labour failed to progress, or was abnormal, the midwives called in the doctor. Because of the current ideas of modesty at that time, he usually had to make his diagnosis without a pelvic examination, or if he performed one, he did it under a sheet! Considering the difficulties, Rigby made a remarkably clear distinction between bleeding that was *inevitable* because the placenta was filling the lower part of the uterus in front of the baby, and the bleeding which occurred *accidentally* because a portion of the placenta separated from its bed on the wall of the uterus.

Today the two types, the inevitable bleeding due to a placenta praevia, and the accidental bleeding of abruptio placentae, still require to be distinguished as treatment is different. The position of the placenta in the uterus can be found by modern equipment, either using ultrasound (see p. 116), or by recording the activity of a special safe radioisotope injected into an arm vein. The substance mixes with the blood, and as the placenta has a good blood supply, its activity is most marked over that part of the uterus in which the placenta lies. The activity is measured with a Geiger counter, and the number of 'bleeps' recorded on a chart (Fig. **17/1**). An expectant mother who is diagnosed as having a placenta praevia remains in hospital until the pregnancy has reached the end of the 37th week. This is called 'expectant treatment', and is used so that the baby may grow in the uterus rather than having to cope with life in a premature nursery. At the 37th week, a decision is made by the doctor whether it is safer for the expectant mother to be delivered normally or by Caesarean section. Four patients in every 10 can deliver normally, and 6 in every 10 who have a placenta praevia require to be delivered by Caesarean section.

Abruptio placentae, the other main condition which causes bleeding in the second half of pregnancy, is of two kinds. In most cases the amount of separation of the placenta is slight, and the pregnancy can safely continue. In a few cases – no more than one-quarter of all – the amount that the placenta separates is greater. In these cases the expectant mother may lose a good deal of blood. Because of this, the doctor gives blood transfusions and brings on labour by breaking the bag of waters. Unfortunately, in the severe forms very few babies survive. However, as the condition usually

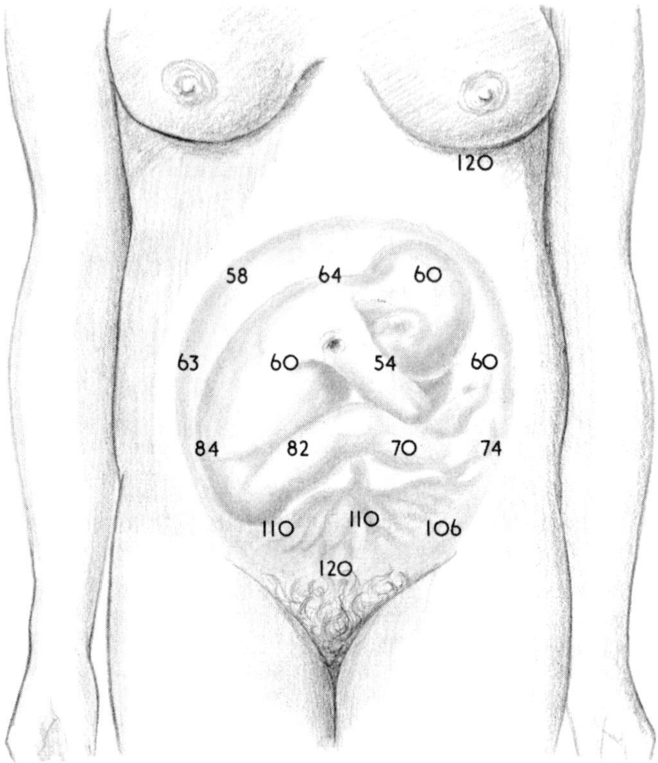

FIG. 17/1. The diagnosis of a placenta praevia by radio-isotopes. The placenta lay under the area of the highest count of 'bleeps'. This was proved at Caesarean section, a live boy being born.

only occurs in women who have previously had several children, the loss of the child does not cause so much grief as would the loss of a first baby.

SWELLING OF THE FINGERS OR FACE

In the second half of pregnancy, for reasons which are unknown, a condition may arise which is called 'toxaemia of pregnancy'. The name is a bad one for there is no toxin, but it has the advantage of being a shorthand reference to three symptoms or signs. These are oedema of the fingers, face or legs; a rise in blood pressure; and the appearance of protein in the urine. Although some swelling of the legs towards evening is normal in pregnancy, swelling of the legs present in the morning, or of the hands or face at any time, is a danger sign. Oedema can be detected by observing if the shoes are uncomfortable, or if the wedding ring is tight. It can also be anticipated by checking if a rapid gain in weight has occurred, and it may be remembered that a weight gain of more than 1 kg. (2 lb.) per week in the second half of pregnancy is a warning of impending 'toxaemia'. A more serious warning is blurring of vision or severe headaches, particularly if associated with oedema.

'Toxaemia of pregnancy' affects about 12 per cent of primigravidae and 6 per cent of multigravidae, but if detected early and treated properly is without danger to mother or child. After childbirth, it disappears rapidly, leaving no trace behind. But if it is neglected, serious complications such as convulsions or 'fits', and the death of the baby can result. This condition is called 'eclampsia'. The expectant mother can understand, therefore, the insistence made by the doctor for regular antenatal visits, when the blood pressure is estimated, the weight gain noted, oedema looked for, and the urine examined. She can also appreciate why she must follow her doctor's instructions implicitly should a rise in blood pressure or other signs of 'toxaemia of pregnancy' occur. The instructions may be simple, such as restricting the diet, particularly the amount of salt used; taking diuretic tablets for a short period to get rid of the excess water (and salt) which the expectant mother has retained; and by increased rest periods at home. Or the doctor may ask her to be admitted to hospital, even when she feels she is quite well. In hospital she will be given sedative drugs. and the doctors and nurses will observe very closely her blood pressure. her weight gain (or one hopes loss), 'fluid balance' (that is, the amount of fluids drunk against the quantity of urine passed), and the growth of the baby. The aim of the medical attendants is to control the 'toxaemia of pregnancy', so that the baby may grow and eventually be born unharmed.

A 'GUSH' OF WATER FROM THE VAGINA

A 'gush' of water from the vagina after the 28th week of pregnancy usually indicates that the bag of membranes, or amniotic sac, has burst. This is called 'rupture of the membranes' by doctors. As will be recalled, the baby grows in the amniotic sac which is filled with amniotic fluid, and the gush of water is the escape of the fluid. If rupture of the membranes occurs, the patient should at once go to hospital. In hospital treatment will depend on how far advanced the pregnancy is. Should this be less than 36 weeks, in all probability the doctor will give sedative drugs in the hope that labour will not start; but if the pregnancy has advanced beyond 36 weeks, he will generally give a drug which stimulates the uterus to contract. The reason is that after the 36th week, the baby is sufficiently mature to survive outside, and there is a slight risk that it may become infected if left in the uterus.

OBSTETRIC OPERATIONS

Women are often most anxious because their friends–if you can call them friends–or neighbours have given them lurid descriptions of the operations they had in their pregnancy. Not only are these descriptions lurid, they are misleading.

Induction of labour

For several reasons, such as 'toxaemia of pregnancy', haemorrhage in pregnancy, Rhesus problems, or pregnancy which has become prolonged to more than 42 weeks, the obstetrician may decide that it is best to induce labour. The usual way in which this is done is to rupture or 'cut' the bag of waters just inside the cervix. The procedure is quite painless, although rather inelegant. The expectant mother is put on an obstetric bed with her feet in stirrups (Fig. **17/2**). The vulva is cleaned, antiseptic lubricant is poured into the vagina, and the doctor makes a pelvic examination. In this, he feels the cervix and notes whether it is soft or not, and how wide open it is. If it is 'suitable', that is soft and at least one finger dilated, he will go ahead and rupture the membranes. This is done with a small

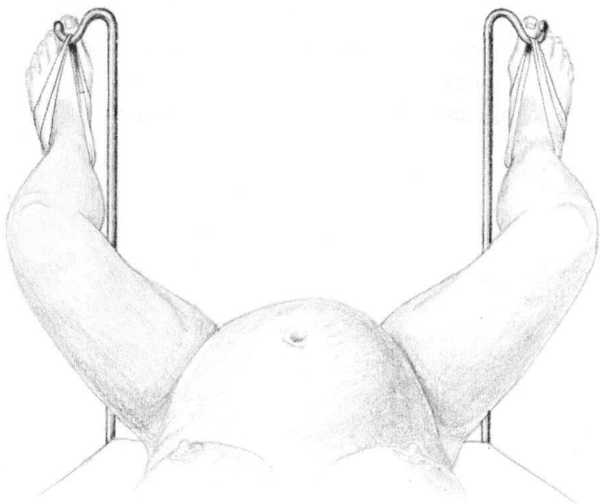

FIG. 17/2. The position in which the mother is placed for certain obstetric manipulations.

instrument, which tears a hole in the bag so that the water runs out. The mother can feel the warm amniotic fluid running down her vagina.

Labour usually starts quite quickly, and the doctor may encourage it to start by setting up a drip into an arm vein of the mother, and carefully running in a drug (oxytocin), which stimulates the uterus to contract. He may decide to give the oxytocin as tablets, which the mother puts in her cheek pouch and allows to dissolve, although this method is not quite as satisfactory as the intravenous drip. With either method, over 95 per cent of women have delivered their baby within 24 hours of the induction.

In the past, pariicularly in England, labour was induced by giving the expectant mother a large dose of castor oil, making her soak in a hot bath, and giving her a large enema. This barbaric, uncouth practice has now ceased, except in isolated, backward areas. It was unkind to the patient, messy for the nurse, and pretty inefficient in starting labour.

Caesarean section

The operation of Caesarean section has nothing to do with Julius Caesar. The word derives from the Latin *caedere*, to cut, for that is what is done. If for some reason the baby cannot be born through the birth-canal, an incision is made in the lower part of the abdominal wall and through the lower part of the uterus. The child is removed through the incisions, which are then carefully repaired with stitches. The mother is anaesthetised throughout the whole operation, and wakes up to hear her baby crying. In the past 30 years, the incidence of Caesarean section has increased considerably. Much of this increase is justified; but some inexcusable, either because the patient demands the operation, or the doctor takes the 'easy way out'. In Australia and Britain, the incidence is about 2 to 4 per cent; in the U.S.A. it seems to be about 5 to 9 per cent.

Part of the reason for the higher rate in the U.S.A. is that there most obstetricians believe that once a Caesarean section has been performed on a patient, all subsequent deliveries should be by Caesarean section. A few take a different view, and believe that many women who have previously been delivered by Caesarean section can be delivered vaginally as safely and with less discomfort in a subsequent pregnancy. This opinion is shared by obstetricians in Australia, Britain and most other countries. In a very careful study in Britain, Sir John Peel (the Queen's Obstetrician) found that 45 per cent of women who had previously had a Caesarean section were delivered vaginally with safety in a subsequent pregnancy, and similar proportions have been obtained in Australia and Malaysia.

So 'once a Caesarean, always a Caesarean' is no longer valid, and an expectant mother whose first baby was delivered by Caesarean section has a 50:50 chance of delivering her next baby vaginally. The only stipulation upon which all obstetricians agree is that a patient who has previously had a Caesarean section must be looked after by a specialist obstetrician, and have her baby in a properly equipped hospital.

Forceps deliveries

In July 1569–400 years ago–a family of Huguenot refugees called

Chamberlen fled from France and arrived in England. One son, Peter, was about 6 years old, and two more sons were to be born subsequently in England, one of them also being called Peter. Although this may not have led to confusion within the family, it has led to the confusion of medical historians, for both Peters became doctors, and one of them invented a secret instrument for the help of women in labour. The elder Peter had a dramatic rise to fame, attended Queen Anne for her confinements, and it is thought that he was the inventor. The Chamberlens kept their secret most successfully, and it is said that when asked to help in a difficult labour, one of them would arrive at the bedside, sit in front of the patient, and have a sheet stretched from the abdomen of the patient and tied round his neck. In the obscurity of the sheet, he would draw a bundle from the pocket of his coat, and manipulations were seen to move the sheet; but the secret instrument was never glimpsed. It was in fact the first obstetric forceps. Chamberlen's forceps were like a pair of outsize sugar tongs, made of metal and covered with leather. He introduced them into the vagina, applied them to the side of the baby's head, and pulled. Sometimes he was successful in delivering the baby, other times not. But successful or not, the family kept the secret for over 100 years, son succeeding father. In about 1670, the grandnephew of the first Peter was in charge, and was tempted to sell his instrument. Hugh Chamberlen offered it for sale for £1,000, a very considerable sum of money in those days. He was invited to go to Paris and demonstrate the value of his instrument. The patient chosen was a dwarf, who had severe rickets, and who had been in labour for days. Chamberlen demanded that he be given a private room, and that no one should observe him at work. He struggled for three hours but failed to deliver the patient, as might be expected. His offer of sale was rejected, but six months later he was in Paris trying again. Finally in 1728, the male line became extinct, and 30 years later the secret instrument was sold and its design made public.

Since that time many changes in the design of the obstetric forceps have made it a precision-tooled, correctly constructed instrument. Over the years, too, the indications in which the forceps are needed, and for which they can be used with safety, have been identified. Doctors who propose to practise obstetrics learn how to handle the instrument, or more correctly the instruments, for today each blade of the forceps is separate. Each blade is inserted into the vagina separately, so that it lies over the side of the baby's head, and once both are in position, the handles of the blades are crossed and joined together at a lock (Fig. **17/3**). In this way the least possible damage is done to the mother or to the baby.

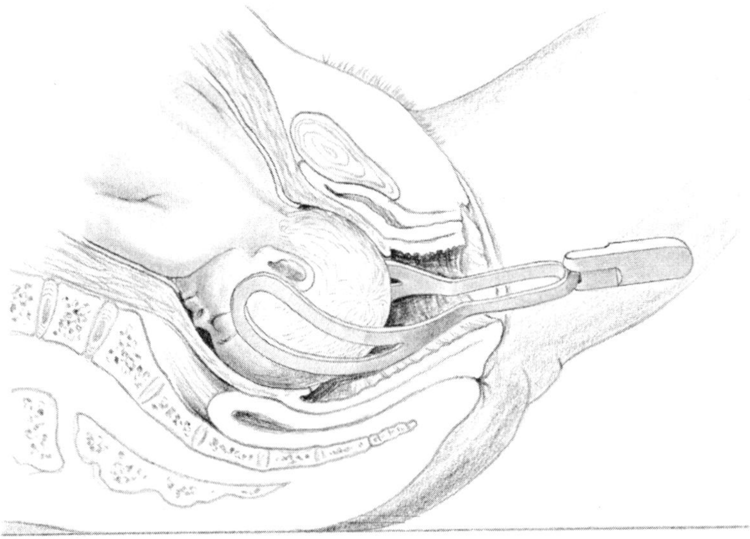

FIG. 17/3. The obstetric forceps. The mother has received a local anaesthetic, and the forceps fit snugly along the sides of the baby's head, like sugar tongs fit along a lump of sugar.

The percentage of mothers on whom forceps are used to effect delivery of the baby varies. In Asia about 1 per cent, in Britain about 6 per cent and in Australia about 12 per cent of the mothers are delivered by forceps; whilst in the U.S.A. the rate exceeds 30 per cent. This is because women in labour in America are very heavily sedated, and often are given an anaesthetic so that they are unable to help in pushing the baby into the world. It is a matter of custom, but even in the U.S.A. most obstetricians are realizing that the more natural childbirth is made, the better it is for mother and for baby.

If forceps are required, the mother can be assured that the

operation will be quite painless. Either a local anaesthetic is given, or else an injection is administered into her spine, called an epidural anaesthetic. The forceps are only inserted into her vagina when the anaesthetic has taken effect. The baby may be born with red marks along the sides of its face corresponding to the shape of the forceps blades. The mother can rest assured that the marks will disappear rapidly.

'Taking the baby with instruments' is still regarded as a serious step by many expectant mothers. Years ago it was, but today with skilled doctors and well-made precision instruments, forceps deliveries are safe. By far the majority of forceps deliveries are made to help the head of the baby over the mother's perineum. This is called a low forceps delivery. In a few cases the baby's head may fail to advance in the second stage of labour, despite strong contractions and good 'pushes' by the mother. If the second stage lasts for more than one and a half hours, the doctor usually introduces the forceps and delivers the baby. This is termed a 'mid-forceps delivery', and it requires far more skill and experience than the low forceps delivery, which is really quite easy. It is usual for the doctor to make a deliberate cut in the perineum with a pair of scissors before delivering the baby. This prevents the tissues from tearing, and it is termed an 'episiotomy'. After the birth of the baby and the placenta, the episiotomy is stitched (see page 201). If the stitching is done properly, it is no more than slightly painful and uncomfortable for two days or so, and with one method of stitching it is virtually painless.

In the last 10 years, an instrument has been suggested which might replace many forceps deliveries. Actually it was originally invented 120 years ago by a famous Scottish obstetrician, Sir James Simpson, who also first used anaesthesia in childbirth. The instrument consists of a flat cap, about 7.5 cm. (3 in.) in diameter. This is connected to a vacuum apparatus. The cup is pushed against the head of the baby, and a vacuum created, so that it is held firmly against the scalp by the atmospheric pressure. The doctor then pulls on the tubing which connects the cup to the vacuum bottle, and the baby is delivered (Fig. **17/4**). The apparatus, called a ventouse, is simple to use, and is said to have the advantage that less is introduced into the vagina than when forceps are used. Because of this, damage to the mother's tissues is less likely to occur.

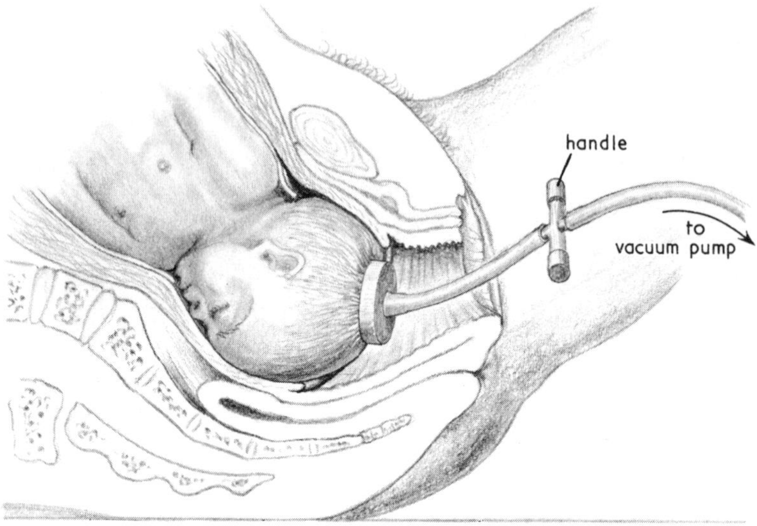

FIG. 17/4. The 'vacuum extractor'. In place of forceps, a small suction cup may be applied to the baby's head, a vacuum created and the baby delivered by pulling on the cup.

It does not really seem to make much difference in most cases whether forceps or a ventouse is used to deliver a baby which is delayed on its journey into the world.

CHAPTER 18

Breasts and breast-feeding

A difference between man and woman which remains obvious despite similar hairstyles and almost identical clothes, is that woman has well-developed breasts. Although the main function of the mammary gland is to provide nourishment for the infant, in vast areas of the world this function has become secondary. The primary function appears to be that the hemispherical swelling of the breast is a potent attraction to males. The ideal of breast beauty varies considerably amongst different races. For example, the Polynesians admire small conical breasts; the Hottentots and North American Indians appear to prefer elongated, melon-shaped, drooping mammary glands; the Chinese women tend to be flat-chested; whilst most European or American men prefer their women to possess large, 'uplifted', hemispherical breasts. The women of the Western world try to please their men as far as they can, and when nature does not provide the appropriate shape and 'uplift', resort to mechanical aids is made, such as brassières, 'falsies', bust-developing creams, exercises and other appliances. The breast-cult of modern man is a recent development, for in the Middle Ages it was considered that: 'The breast of a beautiful woman should be rather broad, and as white as snow or clear as crystal. The breasts must be small, round as a pear or an apple of paradise, and soft as silk to the touch. Large breasts and long hanging breasts are considered ugly.'

Breasts, then, have a functional purpose for milk production to feed the newborn infant, and an erotic function to attract the male. In different cultures and at different times, one or other has predominated.

THE DEVELOPMENT OF THE BREAST

The infantile breast in both sexes consists of a nipple which projects from a pink surrounding area called the *areola*. Around the 10th or 11th year the areola bulges, and the nipple projects from the centre. The development of the male breast ceases at this point, but the female breast develops further as the sex hormones (oestrogen and progesterone) are secreted by the ovaries (Fig. **18/1**). The milk ducts which grow inwards from the nipple, divide into smaller ducts and divide again to form tiny milk-secreting areas called *alveoli*. At the same time fat is deposited around the ducts, so that the breast becomes increasingly protuberant and conical-shaped. After puberty, the development is more rapid, and by the mid-teens the breasts have assumed their adult form, being rounded and firm. In fact, however, they are rarely as round and as firm as our fantasies would have us believe. When a young woman stands up, her breasts hang down slightly, the upper surface is slightly concave and the lower surface slightly convex, joining the skin of the chest at an acute angle. Pregnancy leads to a considerable growth of the ducts and the alveoli, and if the mother breast-feeds her baby, the development is even greater. But in the majority of women the breasts return to their non-pregnant size and shape once lactation has ceased.

The adult breast is of variable size, the size having no relationship to the ability to breast-feed. Small breasts can produce as much milk as large breasts. Anatomically the breast is divided into 15 to 25 sections, called lobes, which are separated from each other by fibrous tissue radiating from the nipple, so that the lobes are rather like the sections of an orange. Each lobe has its own duct system, which ends in a dilated area under the areola and extending into the nipple. This forms a tiny milk reservoir when lactation is established. From this a small duct opens onto the surface of the nipple. There are therefore 15 to 25 openings on the nipple. Going backwards, the main duct divides into smaller ducts, and like the branches of a tree, these ducts divide into still smaller ducts each of which ends in, and drains, a collection of 10 to 100 milk-secreting areas (Fig. **18/2**). The entire duct system is embedded in a pad of fat, and it is this which gives the breast its shape. The duct system of each lobe therefore resembles a tree, the alveoli being the leaves, the small ducts the branches, and the main duct the trunk.

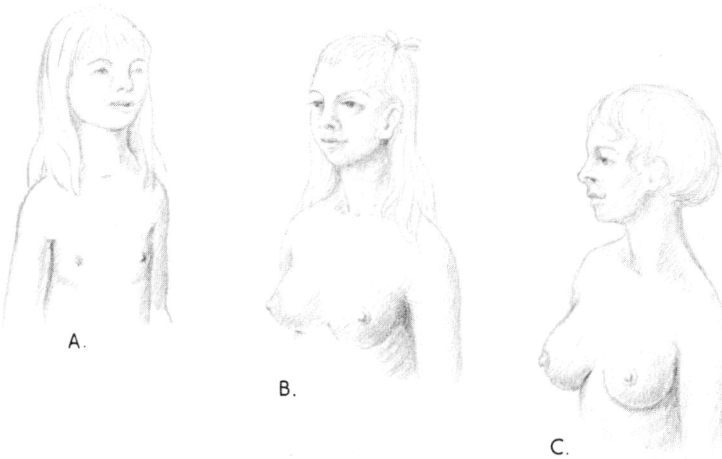

FIG. 18/1. The development of the female breast.
(a) Prepubertal. (b) Late adolescence. (c) Maturity.

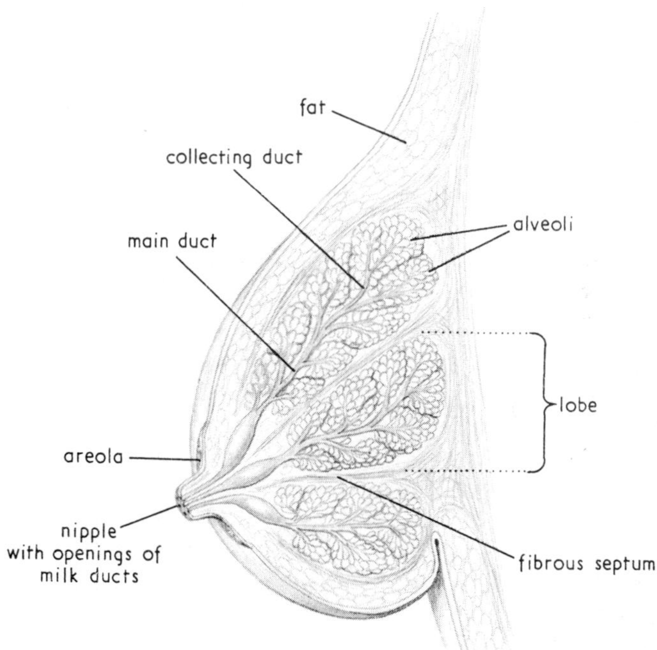

FIG. 18/2. The structure of the breast

During each menstrual cycle, changes occur in the breasts, the ducts developing and the alveoli budding in the second half of the cycle. At the same time fluid oozes into the fatty tissue of the breasts, so that they become firmer and heavier. In some women they may become tender and cause discomfort, which is most marked in the week before menstruation. This is not abnormal, but merely an exaggeration of the normal, and treatment will help. In a few women, the swelling and tenderness persists instead of diminishing during menstruation and disappearing in the first half of the next menstrual cycle. The breasts remain tender and the gland tissue can be felt as irregular lumps. If this occurs, the woman must consult her doctor so that he may investigate fully, and give her treatment to relieve her discomfort.

As the woman becomes older, the breasts tend to get larger and the fibrous tissue bands tend to stretch, so the breasts droop more. After the menopause, the ducts and alveoli become smaller, and the fat starts to go, so that the breasts become smaller, wrinkled and floppy.

IS A BRASSIÈRE REQUIRED?

Modern Western woman is conditioned to wear a brassière. The support has the advantage that it displays the breast more prominently, emphasising its sexual symbolism, and that it prevents premature stretching of the fibrous supports. However, the need for the 'bra' has been exaggerated, and it is probably only really necessary when the breast has become fully mature and hemispherical, during pregnancy and lactation, and if the breasts are very large. It is doubtful if a 'bra' is needed on medical grounds in the teenage years, or by a mature woman who has normal-sized, firm breasts. If a woman feels more comfortable and attractive in a 'bra', then she should wear one; if she is more comfortable and attractive without a 'bra', then she can happily do without. There is little sense though in mothers insisting that their young teenaged daughters require a 'bra': there is no danger of 'drooping', and little to which to give uplift.

In pregnancy, particularly in late pregnancy and during the time a woman breast-feeds her baby, it is advisable to wear a brassière, preferably all the time, both day and night. This is because the increased weight of the breasts at these times may cause stretching of the supporting tissues. The size of the brassière chosen will need to be increased as the breasts grow in pregnancy, and particularly after childbirth. It may be worthwhile buying 'nursing brassières', which have front openings over each nipple and changeable, washable pads to absorb any milk which may leak.

SMALL BREASTS

Because of the strong sexual symbolism of the female breast in Western society, many young adults are concerned if their mammary development fails to equal that of their friends, or more important their favourite film or television star. If the breasts have failed to develop at all, a doctor should be consulted; but if the breasts have developed to some extent and the menstruation has started, there is little that can be done to increase their size. Many women, beguiled by astute advertising, make use of costly oestrogen creams, rubbed assiduously into the breasts. If menstrual function is normal, enough oestrogen is being made by the girl herself and the extra oestrogen will do nothing. Anyhow, oestrogen only causes growth of the ducts of the breasts. What the small-breasted girl lacks is the pad of fat. Nothing, except a better diet, will deposit fat in the breasts. Of course, if the girl has a stooping posture, correction of this and exercises to strengthen the pectoral muscle which lies under the breasts will give them the appearance of being larger by 'throwing' them outwards.

A number of women who have large amounts of money but small amounts of breast tissue seek the attention of plastic surgeons who, for a fee, are prepared to introduce disc-shaped moulds of a plastic material (usually silicone) between the breasts and the pectoral muscles. Obviously, this will make the breasts look larger, although it will not improve their function in any way. The method is not without danger (cancer has followed), and should be avoided in most cases. Certainly a woman should think carefully before deciding to have what is called a mammary prosthesis.

BIG BREASTS

The size of the breasts tends to increase as a woman reaches the age of 35, particularly if she has been pregnant. Most of this enlargement is due to deposition of fat, and although the Western culture approves of large breasts in the young woman, they are not so desirable in later years because instead of being high and firm, they are pendulous and floppy. Exercises are of little help, and although plastic surgery can be performed, it generally only restores the breast temporarily, the enlargement and drooping recurring after a time. And surely a well-designed, well-fitting brassière is preferable to surgery, which will probably only be temporarily successful? However, if the enlargement is gross, surgery may be required.

EXTRA BREASTS

In other mammals more than one breast on each side is normal. In the human, too, a breast (or at least a nipple) can develop anywhere along the breast line, which extends from the armpit to the pubic bone (Fig. **18/3**). The most usual site for the extra breast is in the armpit. The extra breast, which has a nipple, appears as a 'tail' of the normal breast. In a few women nipples are found at other places along the breast line. No treatment is required.

INVERTED NIPPLES

The nipples of the fetus in the womb are normally turned in, or inverted. Usually they evert, or pop-out, in the last weeks of pregnancy, but occasionally they fail to do so. No treatment is required until the woman becomes pregnant. If the nipples fail to evert on their own in pregnancy, and the expectant mother wants to breast-feed, she should make sure that her doctor knows about the nipples and gives treatment. The condition may be so marked that eversion of the nipples and consequently breast-feeding are impossible.

CANCER OF THE BREAST

Cancer of the breast is the most common female cancer. It is twice as common as cancer of the uterus, and 5 women in every 100 can

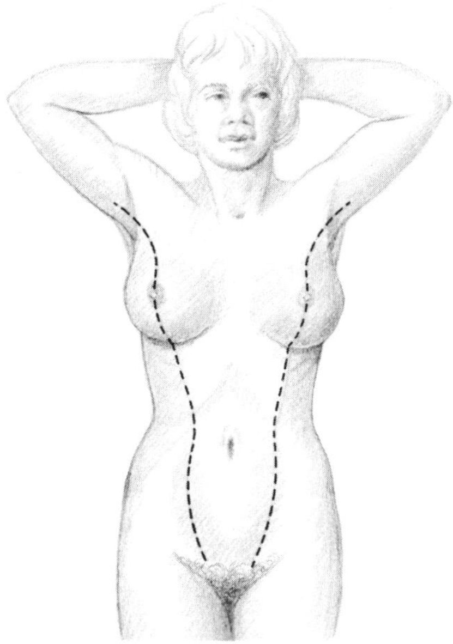

FIG. 18/3. Accessory breasts along the breast line

expect to develop breast cancer in their lifetime. In its late stages, it is virtually incurable; in its early stages, it is usually completely curable.

The only real way to detect breast cancer in its early stages is for the patient herself to routinely examine her breasts, and for her to visit her doctor every year so that he may check that she has not missed a breast cancer. Self-examination of the breasts is not difficult. It should be performed after the menstrual period is over in the younger woman, and once a month in women who have reached the menopause. The woman lies down comfortably, and with the tips of the fingers of the opposite hand palpates each breast in turn, systematically starting at the outer upper part and palpating each section of the breast until she has examined it all. The inner half of the breast is examined with the arm raised (Fig. **18/4A**), and the

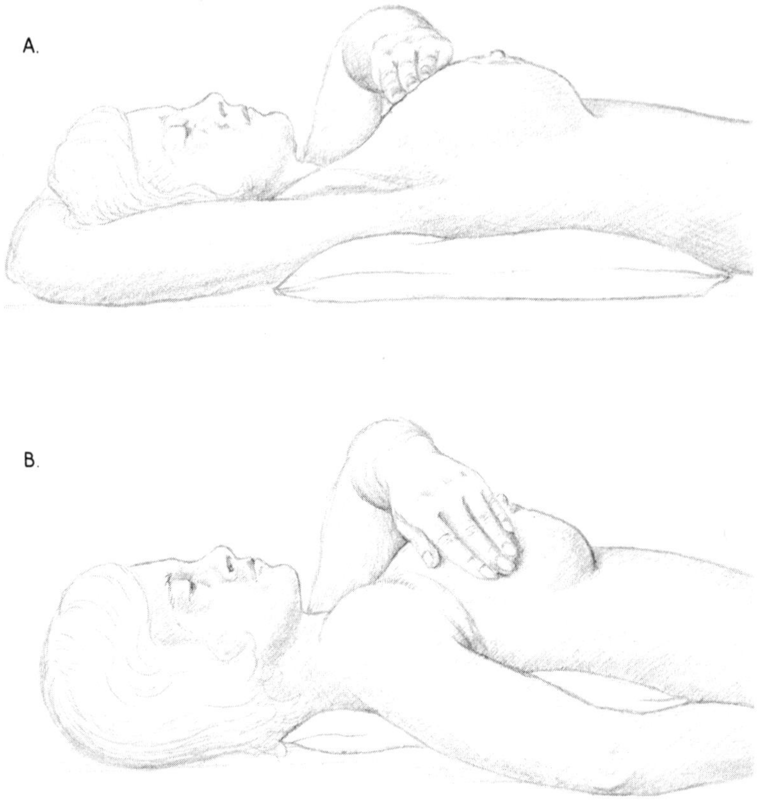

FIG. 18/4. Self-examination of the breasts

outer half with the arm down at the side (Fig. **18/4B**). If the patient palpates a small lump, she should go to her doctor at once. It may not be a cancer, but usually it is necessary to perform a small operation so that the lump can be removed and examined under a microscope.

LACTATION

It is a disturbing fact that fewer and fewer women today breast-feed their babies. In one survey in Cardiff recently, it was found that by the seventh day of the puerperium, only 33 per cent of mothers were giving breast milk to their infants. These findings can be duplicated in many other Western countries. The women in less affluent countries continue to breast-feed their babies, but even in these lands bottle-feeding is gaining ground. Breast-feeding has several very real advantages. Firstly, the milk is sterile, balanced and appropriate to the human baby, just as cat's milk is appropriate for the kitten, bitch's milk is appropriate for the puppy, and cow's milk is appropriate for the calf. Human milk has slightly less protein and casein than cow's milk. The casein is the substance which makes curd. The curd of cow's milk is dense and difficult to digest, in contrast to the light, fluffy curd of human milk. Human milk contains more milk sugar (lactose) than cow's milk, more vitamins and more balanced minerals. In fact 'formula milks' made for bottle-feeding have to be modified from cow's milk by the manufacturers in many complicated ways to make them as much like human milk as possible. Furthermore. 'formula milk' requires care in mixing and in storing to keep it sterile and safe for the baby. Secondly, the act of breast-feeding brings the infant and its mother into a close physical relationship, and the stimulation of the nipple by sucking is pleasant (indeed it has some relationship to sexual stimulation). Not only this, but suckling leads to the release of a hormone from the hypothalamus in the brain, which increases the rapidity and efficiency of involution (or shrinking to normal) of the uterus. Thirdly, and rather facetiously, medical students are taught that the cat cannot get at breast milk and it comes in beautiful containers!

With all the advantages, one would think that all mothers would breast-feed unless there was a medical reason for them to avoid this, yet only one-third do.

The reasons for this distaste for breast-feeding have been studied, but no clear explanation has been found. One factor is that the rigid routine of hospitals, in which the baby is kept in the nursery and only brought to the mother at fixed hours, leads to difficulty in milk production because of restricted suckling. Because of this, and because the baby is obviously hungry, extra feeds using formula milk are given. By this stage, after battling with a fractious infant, a stern nurse and a feeling of failure, the mother's emotions further suppress her own milk production and the baby is put 'on the bottle' completely. In hospitals where babies room-in with their mothers and are fed 'on demand', breast-feeding problems are fewer and more mothers breast-feed. But if the mother has had difficulty with a previous baby leading to failure to breast-feed, the memory may deter her from trying to breast-feed the new infant, and she opts for bottle-feeding at once. Another possible reason for the reduced wish to feed may be linked to parental upbringing of the mother when she was a child. Despite the current display of the breast, despite its sexual symbolism, many mothers instil the belief into their daughters that the breast is a forbidden zone, to be hidden and never exposed. In a study of English mothers, two psychologists reported that 'modesty and a feeling of distaste' formed a major reason for their preference for formula-feeding, and in the U.S.A. another group reported that the mothers they studied were 'repelled' by the idea of giving their breasts to their infants. They were excessively embarrassed at the idea or were too 'modest' to nurse. In other studies of women of higher social groups, reasons for not wanting to feed were that feeding would 'interfere with the mother's social life'; bottle-feeding was so much easier; and breast-feeding would spoil the shape of the mother's breasts. These are selfish reasons, but are nevertheless felt.

If any advice can be given, it should be that for good reasons, breast-feeding is best feeding; but if the mother decides against breast-feeding for whatever reason, the baby will thrive provided the formula milk chosen is a reputable one, and the mother knows how to manage it.

Demand feeding

Many of the difficulties which have deterred a mother from breast-feeding her baby will be eliminated if 'demand feeding' is adopted. This is what mothers have done since mammals evolved, and it is what the majority of the mothers in the world do today. It was rejected in Western countries about 40 years ago for the routine three-hourly or four-hourly feeding, which was more convenient for hospital routine.

Demand feeding implies that the baby is fed when it is hungry, when it demands food. In 'scheduled feeding' the baby is fed at a time decided by the nursing staff, even if this is inconvenient to the mother, and whether the baby is hungry or not. Babies are even woken up to be fed, and, of course, difficulties arise! It is like waking a man at 11 p.m. four hours after he has eaten a steak, and telling him he has to eat another steak! Some can, many cannot.

For demand feeding to be successful, the baby must 'room-in' with its mother. She is in close contact with it at all times, she cuddles it, she plays with it, she notes its changes in mood, she learns when its cry means hunger. From all these visual, tactile and emotional links, messages are carried to her brain, and the complex system which encourages milk secretion and its flow from the alveoli of the breasts to the collecting ducts is initiated. When the baby is hungry, the mother feeds it, changes it, pets it and then sleeps. A baby enjoys the breast, it nuzzles the nipples, its hands grasp the breast; and as it drinks its toes curl sensuously, its fingers move rhythmically, and in male babies erection of the penis is common. The mother notices these signs of contentment, she is relaxed, and a further flow of milk occurs.

In the first three days after childbirth, however, milk flow is minimal. The baby has sufficient reserves for this period, and it is put to the breast merely to encourage the onset of lactation. It should not be put to the breast for too long, or the nipples may become sore; but it can be put for short periods as often as the mother wishes, since it is living beside her.

By the evening of the third day, or the next morning, lactation should have started, the milk should have 'come in', and proper breast-feeding can begin.

The technique of breast-feeding

The most important factor in successful breast-feeding is to be comfortable. It does not much matter whether the mother breast-feeds her baby when sitting up, on her side, or lying down. If she is most comfortable lying down, the baby lies in the bed beside her and she lies on her side facing it. She then adjusts her position so that the baby can nuzzle her nipple and eventually can take the nipple into its mouth. If the baby stuffs it in too far, it may be unable to breathe, and the mother may need to press her breast down from its nose to give him 'air space'.

If she prefers to feed sitting up, she must get comfortable, and often a chair with arms is preferable to one without. She can put a pillow on the arm of the chair, and then has a convenient prop for her arm as she holds her baby. Once again, the baby may need 'air space' when feeding, and she may need to press her breast away from its nose with her fingers.

It is immaterial which position is adopted for breast-feeding, but it is of great importance to make sure that the whole of the areola is inside the baby's mouth. In the diagram on page 249, it can be seen that the duct from each alveolus expands in the areola to form a sinus, or milk reservoir. These storage areas hold the milk, and when the baby squeezes them with its gums, milk spurts out of the nipple and into the baby's mouth. As the baby relaxes its grip to swallow the milk, more milk comes down from the alveoli to fill the sinuses again. In fact, the 'sucking' action made by the baby is only partly responsible for its obtaining milk; the squeezing effect is far more important. Sucking has another purpose, and this is to keep the areola and nipple well within the baby's mouth, and to draw the milk which spurts all over its mouth and into its throat.

If the baby only bites onto the nipple, it will get hardly any milk, will become furious and bite harder. This will give the mother a sore nipple. But if the baby takes the nipple and the areola into its mouth, its gums will grip on the areola, leaving the nipple free, and not damaging it. Should the areola be very large, the mother may have to compress it between her thumb and finger so that the baby can get the nipple well inside its mouth. The mother does not need to hold the baby's head and direct it to the nipple, or to force its mouth open to get the nipple inside; in fact many paediatricians believe that this makes him baffled, bewildered and furious. All she needs to do is to get the baby comfortably nuzzling her nipple. Once the baby wants it, she must make sure the nipple is well inside its mouth, and that it chews on the areola. Nor should she pull the baby off her breast, because it hurts her and annoys the baby. It is easy to detach the baby from the breast, by simply slipping a finger into the corner of its mouth, between its gums, to break the suction.

The schedule of breast-feeding

This has been mentioned already. In the first three days after childbirth, only a thick yellow secretion (called colostrum) is produced, and as the baby has its own reserve stores of food, it is only put to the breast for 3 to 5 minutes, three times in the first 24 hours, and then every 4 hours during the day. The purpose of this is to encourage the milk to 'come in'. Of course, if the baby wakes up and is hungry, the four-hourly routine is replaced by 'demand feeding'.

The milk 'comes in' usually on the 3rd or 4th day, but sometimes later, and either gradually or all at once. By now the baby is hungry and much more wide awake than earlier. It may cry, and the mother who 'rooms-in' with her baby rapidly learns to distinguish the cry of hunger, from the cry of discomfort. The baby is put to the breast, and is given alternate breasts first at alternate feeds. It may get sufficient from one breast, or may need to be put on both at a single feed. Usually, too, the other breast leaks milk when the baby feeds. The baby should never stay on one breast for longer than 12 minutes, as it will have got most of the milk in this time, and if the baby stays on longer the nipple may become sore. If the mother feeds 'on demand', she will generally find it easier than if the baby is fed at fixed times, for the reasons which have already been given. However, with demand feeding, once the milk has 'come in', it is unlikely that the average baby needs to be fed more frequently than every three hours. Fractiousness before this time can be coped with by cuddling, which is probably what the baby wants.

The quantity of milk

It is very difficult to decide from the length of time which the baby spends feeding if it is getting enough milk. As the baby usually gets nearly all the milk available in the first 10 minutes, it may continue to feed because it is comfortable, or because it is getting a little trickle of milk, or because it is asleep. But if the baby is content, it has had enough. Nor can you tell if the baby is satisfied or still hungry by the fact that it cries after a feed. The cry may be due to 'wind', or because the baby is wet, rather than because it is still hungry. Nor can you tell about the quantity (or the quality) of the milk from the fullness of the breasts or the appearance of the milk. In the first week or two the breasts are usually firm, and appear full, although the quantity of milk secreted is not great. After a while, the sequence of production of milk, the 'let down' or passage of milk to the milk sinuses, and the balance between demand and production of milk is established, and the breasts appear less full although in fact milk production has increased.

The best way of telling if there is sufficient milk is observation of the baby. If it is happy, contented and gaining weight (checked every few days, not after every few feeds), there is enough milk. If the baby is fractious but gaining weight, it is getting enough milk but may be guzzling it down too fast and getting 'wind'. Only if the baby is hungry, crying and not gaining weight, need there be any worry, and even then inadequate milk supply is only one possible reason.

One of the most important ways of being sure that there is sufficient milk is to avoid being worried. The young mother who is full of anxiety about her milk supply, and who fusses constantly that her baby is not getting enough, may well reduce the amount of milk she secretes. Worry is a good way to reduce milk supplies! Modern woman relies too much on scales, and on formulae for feeding. In the developing countries of the world, millions of mothers who have no scales feed their babies 'on demand'; the babies seem to thrive, and to get all the milk they need. Incidentally, it is almost impossible to overfeed a baby.

The quality of breast milk

The quality of the breast milk of a mother who has a normal diet is high. There is no such thing as 'weak milk'. If the baby is fractious, it is because it has to work to feed, or because it is being suckled in the wrong way–not because the milk is weak. Generally speaking, what the mother eats or does will not alter the quality of her milk. She can continue to eat all the foods she is accustomed to eating, and she can drink alcohol (in moderation, for a drunk mother is hardly a good mother!), tea or coffee. A few substances do cross into the milk and affect the baby. The most annoying drugs are cascara, which no woman needs, and bromides, which can be avoided. A few mothers find that certain foods also affect their baby, although their friends who are breast-feeding find that their babies are not affected by the same foods. It is obviously a peculiarity confined to that mother and her baby, and the simple answer is to avoid that particular food in the future.

Anxiety about the progress of the baby, nervousness and insecurity can reduce the *quantity* of milk secreted, which makes the baby fractious, but this will not alter the *quality*.

Myths about breast-feeding

A reason given by many mothers–particularly French women–for avoiding breast-feeding is that it will spoil their figures, and cause the breasts to sag. These two statements are untrue. A woman who breast-feeds her baby does not need to stuff herself with food–she has already got a store of fat during pregnancy for this very purpose, which she can burn up. Nor do mothers who feed their babies develop sagging breasts. After a pregnancy the breast is a little more mature and soft, rather than being pointed and firm, but it will not sag, particularly if during the last weeks of pregnancy and during the puerperium the mother wears a well-fitting brassière, day and night.

Another myth is that breast-feeding 'tires out' a mother. Although the care of a new baby does require energy, and consequently the mother should take an increased quantity of milk (for calcium), protein, vegetables and fruit, breast-feeding is probably less tiring than bottle-feeding. In breast-feeding all the mother has to do is put the baby to the breast; if she 'formula feeds', she has to prepare the formula, keep the milk sterile, warm it, feed the baby, clean the bottle, and get the next feed ready. Some women find that they are uncertain how to care for their baby, and worry about the child's progress. These women are apt to feel 'worn out and tired', and blame this on breast-feeding rather than on the disturbed sleep and additional responsibilities which a new baby demands.

The final myth is a particularly insidious one. This is that a woman who fails to breast-feed her baby has failed as a mother. This is quite untrue. Breast-feeding offers the most suitable milk for the baby, and it brings the mother and her baby into a close, intimate contact; but for psychologists to say that the bottle-fed baby is deprived and will be less stable and happy in later life is just stupid. The mother can show her concern for her baby by caring for it as she feeds it with the bottle, and she can cuddle it between feeds. If she fails to breast-feed or decides not to breast-feed, she is not 'depriving her child' and need not feel guilty. Bottle-fed babies cannot be identified from breast-fed babies in later life.

Difficulties of breast-feeding

ENGORGEMENT. If the mother determines to follow the plan of 'demand feeding', it may still be necessary to put the baby to the breast at regular intervals in the first three days. By the 3rd or 4th day of the puerperium, the milk 'comes in'. This means that milk production is now in full swing, but that the passage of milk into the ducts and out of the nipple is not yet properly organized. In some women the breasts become heavy, tense and warm. In a few women they are painful. The breasts are said to be 'engorged'. Engorgement is only temporary, lasting for less than 24 hours, and the doctors and nursing staff are fully competent to help the mother.

CRACKED NIPPLES. In normal feeding, the infant grasps the areola of the nipple, and not the nipple itself. The nipple lies free in the baby's mouth. How it should be grasped can be visualized if you suck your thumb, so that the end is freely movable in the mouth. If the nipple is free within the infant's mouth, its gums compress the small reservoirs in the lower part of the nipples and milk squirts out of the openings in the nipples. If the nipple is not far enough in the baby's mouth, the milk does not flow easily, the baby becomes frustrated and sucks harder. This may cause cracked, painful nipples. Cracked and painful nipples can also be caused by letting the baby suck for too long. Normally the baby empties a breast in under 7 minutes, and it is pointless to permit it to suckle on that breast for more than 12 minutes. If cracked nipples occur, the baby should be taken off the breast for a couple of days, and the breast emptied by manual expression, the expressed milk being sterilized and fed to the baby in a bottle. An antibiotic ointment may be applied to the breast on a doctor's advice.

INSUFFICIENT MILK PRODUCTION. Fear, anxiety, pain, lack of privacy, and unsympathetic attendants can prevent the milk from passing along the ducts within the breast. In these cases, although milk is secreted, the baby gets very little and cries with hunger. This aggravates the anxiety and a vicious circle is set up. Milk production is best in a mother who is healthy, fairly young, has a good diet and who wants to breast-feed. Milk production is likely to be less if the mother is ill, older and poorly motivated about breast-feeding. Milk production may diminish if the mother starts taking oral contraceptives, but this varies considerably.

Various foods and drugs have been recommended to improve milk production, but none has been proved to be of any value. Drinking excessive water or milk does not improve milk production, nor does the use of iodine drops, special 'lactation foods', or thyroid tablets. The most efficient way of establishing a good milk flow is a knowledge of how milk is produced; a desire to breast-feed; a healthy, hungry baby; and sympathetic, helpful nurses.

MENSTRUATION AND LACTATION. This matter is discussed on p. 219.

MASTITIS. Occasionally infection enters the lactating breast, usually introduced through cracked nipples, during the second or third week of the puerperium. The breasts become engorged, hard, reddened, tender and painful. If this happens, breast-feeding should be stopped, temporarily at least, and the mother should visit her doctor.

CHAPTER 19

The things that happen to women

During life it is inevitable that a woman will have her share of anxiety, of illness, of strain, as well as her share of satisfaction and happiness. But because she is biologically different from man, she may develop conditions unique to woman. Many of these are minor, but require attention. In most instances a woman should consult her doctor, but as doctors are busy men and all too often do not explain adequately to the patient the nature of the condition from which she is suffering, she often remains anxious. This chapter attempts to redress this, and to give a woman the chance of understanding herself better. There is no doubt that fear of the unknown is a potent factor in aggravating disease, and insight into the nature of a disorder is a major step to its cure. For convenience, the conditions which may affect a woman in her reproductive years are considered in as alphabetical an order as is practicable.

ENLARGEMENT OF THE WOMB

The most common cause of enlargement of the womb is pregnancy! But sometimes the womb is enlarged by a muscle tumour, or because of the effects of anxiety.

The muscle tumours are called myomata or 'fibroids'. For some unknown reason, one or more of the muscle fibres which make up the uterus start developing, and quite soon a few small pea-sized tumours appear deep in the muscle wall of the uterus. At this stage no one can detect them, but as the months or years pass–for they grow very slowly–the tumours become the size of a golf ball, a tennis ball or even of a grapefruit. By this time the patient can feel a lump in her abdomen, or if the tumour has grown inwards and distorted the shape of the cavity of the uterus, she may have heavier or irregular menstrual periods. Usually she goes to her doctor, who performs a pelvic examination and can tell from this if there is a single fibroid, or if the womb is misshapen and enlarged by several fibroid tumours. It is unusual for a woman who has children early in life to develop fibroids, and the tumours are more likely to found in spinsters, or women who have children late in life, which has led to the saying that 'fibroids develop in a disappointed womb'. The tumours are very common, and more than 20 per cent of women have fibroids in their womb. In many cases no treatment is required, as the tumour is not causing any symptoms, but in the few women who have symptoms, treatment is needed. The treatment chosen depends upon the patient's age and her desire to have further children.

If a youngish woman, who is anxious to have children, is found to have fibroids which are causing symptoms, the doctor can often operate to remove the fibroids and leave the uterus. It is a bit like a complicated shelling of peas, and although there is a slight chance that the fibroids may grow again, the chances of pregnancy are good. In an older woman, or a woman who wants no further children, the operation chosen is usually that of hysterectomy, in which the womb is removed.

Another cause of enlargement of the womb is anxiety. The ancient Greeks believed that a woman's emotions were made in her womb. The Greek word for womb is *hysteros*–which is why women were said to be hysterical. Of course, the place in which the emotions occur is the brain, but if the emotions–whether due to anxiety, frustration or unhappiness–operate for a sufficient time, they cause a smooth enlargement of the womb, and heavy periods. All too often, doctors have mistaken this emotionally-stimulated enlargement of the womb for fibroids, and have performed a hysterectomy. This cured the heavy periods, but the disturbed emotions were unaltered, and other disorders (usually unexplained abdominal pain or backache) appeared 3 to 6 months after the operation. Occasionally a surgical operation is needed to cure the condition (which is called myohyperplasia), but in most cases what is needed is sympathetic understanding and perhaps some drugs to help temporarily.

ENDOMETRIOSIS

Endometriosis is a strange disorder, which affects spinsters and infertile married women more often than those fertile women who have children early in the reproductive years. The term means that the pieces of the lining of the womb (the endometrium) either form small nests (or cysts) in the muscle of the womb (which will, of course, then become bigger), in the ovaries, or in other parts of the pelvis. These nests of endometrium act like miniature wombs, and at the time of menstruation a tiny amount of bleeding occurs. Since the blood cannot escape, the cyst is stretched and becomes painful. The woman complains of dysmenorrhoea, which increases during menstruation and is worse on the last day. If a cyst has formed in the pelvis behind the womb, as sometimes happens, sexual intercourse can be painful when the husband's penis is moving deeply inside the vagina. Because of dysmenorrhoea, painful sexual intercourse, or failure to become pregnant, the woman attends her doctor. In the past the only treatment was surgery, but today hormone treatment using drugs like those contained in the Pill can cure the condition, and enable the patient to conceive if she so wishes. Some women do need surgery, but often all the gynaecologist has to do is to make a tiny incision below the umbilicus and introduce an instrument, rather like a periscope, so that he can see the extent of the disease. This minor operation is done under anaesthesia and is painless. Once the doctor knows how much the endometriosis has involved the genital organs, he can decide if surgery or hormone treatment is best, or if both are needed.

HYSTERECTOMY

One of the most common surgical operations performed on women is removal of the womb, or hysterectomy. In fact, many doctors believe that the operation is done too often for too little reason. An American surgeon has written that a woman has about 1,000 dollars-worth of 'expendable parts', a major one being her womb, and by the age of 50 has had most of them removed! This is perhaps extreme, for in many cases a well-performed hysterectomy can cure a patient who was previously miserable. But, even so, the operation is still done too often, for too little reason, and without explaining to the patient its effects. It is usual if the woman is under the age of 45, and often whatever her age, to leave the ovaries in place, so that they can continue to function and secrete the female sex hormones. If this is done, and the gynaecologist is skilful, the only after-effect of a hysterectomy is that menstruation ceases and pregnancy cannot possibly occur. Hysterectomy does not make a wife sexually mutilated and undesirable; it does not shorten her vagina so that sexual intercourse is impossible or potentially dangerous; it does not lead to obesity. The opposite is still widely believed, however, and is untrue. Firstly, a woman is sexually desirable because of her character and personality, and her feminine attributes are in part due to these and in part to the oestrogen secreted by the ovaries. Provided the ovaries have not been removed, and are still functioning, she will not become an 'old woman', unwanted and undesirable. If for any reason the gynaecologist has to remove a young woman's ovaries, he will make sure that she is given oestrogen tablets. Secondly, after hysterectomy the vagina is not shortened; in fact if anything it is longer. When the womb is removed, the vagina has to be cut at its uppermost end, and the cervix no longer projects into it (Fig. **19/1**). Once the cut has healed strongly, which takes about six weeks, sexual intercourse can be resumed safely and with normal satisfaction. Since the womb has been removed, pregnancy cannot occur and no contraceptive measures are needed. Thirdly, hysterectomy is not followed by obesity, unless the woman takes no exercise after the operation and spends her time eating. If she does this, of course she will get fat.

MENSTRUAL DISORDERS

Because of the complicated control of menstruation which was described in Chapter 4, and because of the impact of the emotions upon the controlling area in the brain, it can be readily understood that from time to time during a woman's life menstrual disorders may occur. These are, in general, of three kinds: the menstrual periods may occur less frequently, or cease altogether; they may occur regularly but be very heavy; or they may become quite irregular in time of onset, in their duration and in the amount of blood lost. These irregularities are more usual before the age of 20 and after the age of 35, but may occur at any time during the reproductive

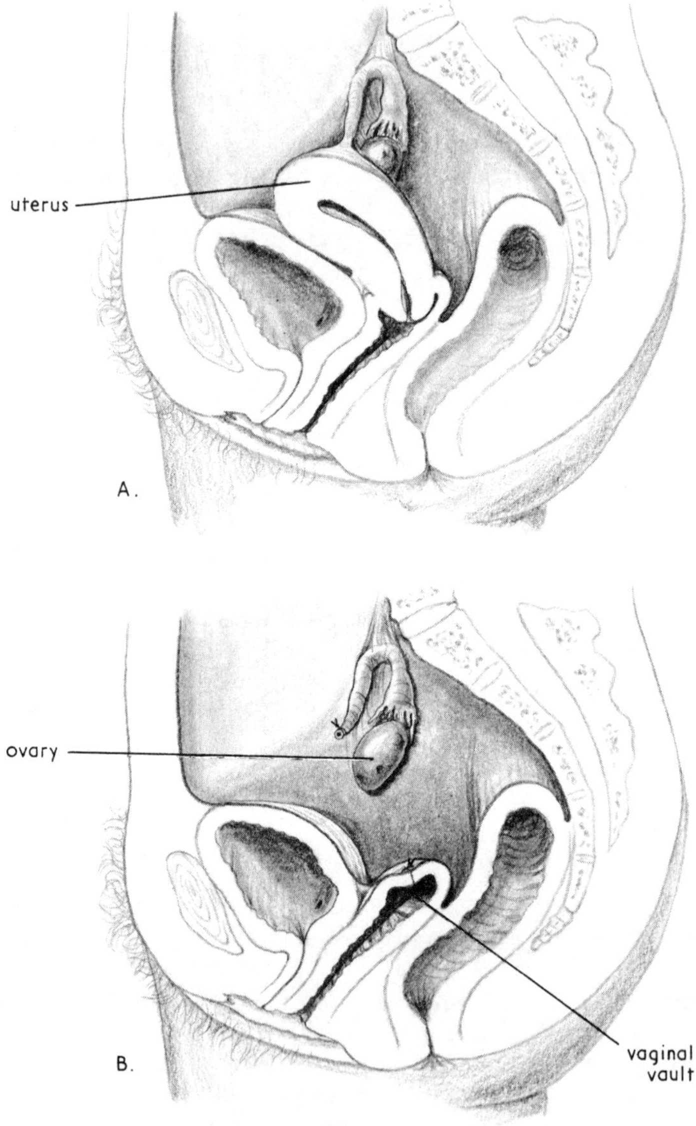

FIG. 19/1. The length of the vagina shown in A is not shortened by hysterectomy shown in B

years. Furthermore, many women find that the character of their menstrual period alters during the reproductive years. Often the periods become heavier for a while after childbirth, and as the age of 40 is approached.

A reduction in the amount of blood lost during menstruation, a longer interval between periods, or the absence of periods (amenorrhoea) can cause concern. There may be an underlying disorder of hormone secretion, or the woman who has amenorrhoea may be pregnant. However, pregnancy is not the only cause, although it is by far the commonest. Amenorrhoea sometimes occurs if a girl leaves home to take up a job in a different environment, or if she is under great emotional stress. In the War years, women interned by the Japanese under primitive, unfamiliar conditions, noticed that their periods ceased soon after internment; and today some women find that their menstrual periods cease during bereavement after the death of a loved one. The problem can usually be resolved by consulting a doctor, who may require to do certain tests.

Irregular or heavy menstrual periods can either mean that a disease is present in the uterus or ovaries, or can be due to an emotional disturbance affecting the hormonal control of menstruation, which is the more common cause. The real reason can only be determined after a careful medical examination, which usually includes a diagnostic curettage (or 'cleaning' of the lining of the womb). This minor operation is performed under an anaesthetic, but the patient needs to spend only the day in hospital, and does not really need to have her pubic hair shaved. The lining of the womb is 'scraped' or 'cleaned' using an instrument called a curette, which is introduced into the uterus through the cervix. The pieces of the lining of the womb are then collected and sent to a laboratory, so that the exact diagnosis of the cause of the bleeding can be made. This is why the operation should be called a *diagnostic* curettage, although it is loosely known as a 'd. and c.'. Not every patient needs to have the operation, but if she is over the age of 35 it is usually performed, as irregular bleeding may be the first sign of cancer of the womb, although this is a rare cause of irregular bleeding at least in the years before the 'change of life'. Any bleeding from the womb which occurs *after* the 'change of life' is possibly due to cancer, and a diagnostic curettage is essential.

In years past, irregular or heavy bleeding was treated by hysterectomy provided that the woman wanted no further children. Today the potent sex hormones do the job just as well, and avoid the necessity of an operation, for many women at least. However, hysterectomy is still needed in certain cases. The decision is best made by a gynaecologist in consultation with the patient's family doctor who knows about her background. To repeat what I have written, too many hysterectomies are still being performed for too little, or the wrong, reason.

OBESITY

Women are never satisfied. They are either too thin and want to be fatter, or too fat and want to be thinner. Those who are too fat for their height are called obese. The average weight for height is shown in Table **19/1**, so you can calculate if you are overweight, or obese. Of course, you may not need to calculate; it may be obvious to your friends and yourself that you are too fat. Obesity is to some extent dependent on a woman's body structure and metabolism. If she comes from an obese family and has obese parents, she is likely to become obese no matter how hard she tries to avoid it. Many women find it infuriating that some of their friends can eat and drink as much as they like and never put on weight, whilst they themselves appear to gain weight merely by looking at food. Looking at food does not put on weight. Eating does, and within the limits established by heredity, fat women are fat because they eat too much and eat the wrong foods. Women who are too fat can lose weight, but it is a slow process and requires great self-control, discipline and persistence.

Because of woman's desire to be something other than she is, and in particular to be thinner, an infinite variety of diets, drugs, regimens, exercises, cures, massages, hydrotherapy and quackery constantly are being recommended. The propagators of these methods have grown rich, a few women have grown thin, but many have not changed; and it is these women who keep the diet-propagators rich, as they in desperation try new methods and adopt other gimmicks. Hardly a week passes without a woman's magazine advising their readers to try this 'six-day tripe diet', or that 'four-day egg and anchovy diet', or the other 'orange, onions and oyster diet'.

It needs to be repeated, a woman can lose weight if she has self-

Table 19/1

Desirable Weight (Pounds)

*Women (Age 25 and over)**				
Height Feet	*Inches*	*Small Frame*	*Medium Frame*	*Large Frame*
4	8	92– 98	96–107	104–119
4	9	94–101	98–110	106–122
4	10	96–104	101–113	109–125
4	11	99–107	104–116	112–128
5	0	102–110	107–119	115–131
5	1	105–113	110–122	118–134
5	2	108–116	113–126	121–138
5	3	111–119	116–130	125–142
5	4	114–123	120–135	129–146
5	5	118–127	124–139	133–150
5	6	121–131	128–143	137–154
5	7	126–135	132–147	141–158
5	8	130–140	136–151	145–163
5	9	134–144	140–155	149–168
5	10	138–148	144–159	153–173

*For girls between 18 and 25, subtract 1 pound for each year under 25.

control, discipline, persistence and only eats the right foods–and they are many.

If a woman really wants to lose weight, she has to stick to the diet and obey the rules. Drugs do not cause weight loss, although they may act as a 'prop' to make the hardships of the diet less. One of the most commonly used drugs is amphetamine, which should be avoided because it is an addictive drug. It is far safer to have self-discipline than to use drugs, and the end results are better. Women who use drugs as well as a reducing diet have a much higher chance of putting on weight again later. The woman who sticks to her diet until she has reduced to her desired or 'ideal' weight, without needing drugs, finds it far easier to keep on a diet which will maintain her at that weight. The 'ideal' weight for height and body build is shown in Table **19/1**. These weights are of women wearing thin underclothes ('bra' and panties).

Problems may arise when dining out. I know that it might be difficult and impolite to refuse some special, but fattening dish which your hostess has gone to a great deal of trouble to prepare. The solution is to accept a small portion, and to try to eat less earlier in the day before attending the dinner. If pre-dinner drinks are served, take either soda-water or a single whisky and water. At dinner try to have no more than one glass of wine.

In Table **19/2** you can see the foods you may not eat, the foods which are rationed, and the foods of which you may eat all you wish, within reason, of course! It is doubtful, for example, if you will eat more than 240 g., that is 8 oz., of meat, or more than 4 eggs a day! Table **19/3** gives an example of a diet for one week, but of course you can make up your own if you wish.

Table 19/2

Foods you may not eat

Fried foods.
Sugar, jam, marmalade or honey.
Sweets or chocolates.
Nuts.
Butter (beyond the ration of $\frac{1}{2}$ oz.), margarine, fat or oil.
Bread (except in the ration, see below), cake, biscuits, toast or breakfast cereals.
Macaroni, spaghetti or semolina.
Rice (except boiled and replacing the potato ration).
Puddings, ice-cream, dried or tinned fruits.
Cream.
Alcohol.

Foods of which you may eat as much as you like (within reason!)

Lean meat, poultry, game, rabbit, liver, kidney, sweetbreads (provided you do not use flour, breadcrumbs or thick sauces).
Fish, steamed, boiled or grilled only.
Eggs.

Vegetables of all kinds–fresh, frozen, dried or tinned (except for baked beans, lima beans, kidney beans, sweet corn, lentils, avocado, sweet potatoes, which are all prohibited).

Salads, tomatoes, cucumbers, beetroot, watercress or parsley (together more than one of these makes a 'combination salad'), but only without oil or mayonnaise, although you can use a lemon and vinegar dressing if you wish.

Fresh fruit, grapefruit, cranberries, strawberries, melon (but only *one* apple, orange, peach or banana if this is chosen to replace the fruits listed).

Soup, clear such as consommé, broth, 'meat extract'.

Salt, pepper, mustard, Worcester sauce for seasoning (but no other sauces).

Saccharin, if desired for sweetening.

Tea, coffee (milk can be added from the ration).

Foods which are rationed

Bread –3 slices weighing 30g., or 1 oz., each. Wholemeal bread is preferable to white bread.

Butter –$\frac{1}{2}$ oz.

Milk –300 ml., 10 fluid oz., of whole milk, *or* 600 ml., 20 fluid oz., of skimmed milk or yoghurt.

Potato–boiled, steamed or baked 'in the skin'; but not fried, 'chipped' or roasted. A maximum of 240 g. (8 oz.) can be eaten.

or Rice –120 g. (4 oz.) can be substituted for the potato.

Table 19/3

A Recommended Diet

(giving approximately 1,600 calories a day)

BREAKFAST Every day you may choose from grapefruit (a half), strawberries, or a slice of melon; then eat an egg or grilled tomatoes and mushrooms, with one or two slices of bread or toast only; tea or coffee, with milk from the ration.

MONDAY	*Lunch*	Clear soup Egg salad 1 slice of bread Coffee or tea
	Dinner	Steak, tomatoes, celery, green salad, baked potato Apple Coffee or tea
TUESDAY	*Lunch*	Grilled kidneys on toast (1 slice) An apple, an orange or a banana
	Dinner	Boiled chicken, fresh beans, baked potato Grapefruit ($\frac{1}{2}$ fresh) Coffee or tea
WEDNESDAY	*Lunch*	Egg and combination salad, 1 potato, boiled or baked in skin
	Dinner	Consommé 2 lamb chops (cut off the fat before grilling), peas, baked potato Coffee or tea
THURSDAY	*Lunch*	Eggs (grilled), mashed potato, spinach or cauliflower Orange, apple or grapefruit
	Dinner	Steak, salad, 1 baked potato Fresh fruit Coffee or tea
FRIDAY	*Lunch*	Poached eggs and spinach 1 slice of bread or toast Coffee or tea
	Dinner	Consommé Fish, baked potato, courgettes (zucchini) or carrots Fruit Coffee or tea

SATURDAY	*Lunch*	Egg, salad, celery 1 slice of wholemeal bread Coffee or tea
	Dinner	Boiled chicken and rice, mushrooms, marrow (summer squash) Melon Coffee or tea
SUNDAY	*Lunch*	Sweetbreads or eggs with mushrooms, combination salad 1 slice of wholemeal bread Fruit Coffee or tea
	Dinner	Vegetable soup Steak, combination salad, baked potato Fruit–orange or apple Coffee or tea

There is no instant method of losing weight. It takes time and discipline. If a woman is 14 lb. (6 kg.) over-weight, for example, she can calculate that 12 lb. of this is due to excess fat and perhaps 2 lb. to water retention. Twelve pounds of fat contain about 50,000 calories. The normal, averagely-active woman needs about 2,100 calories a day, and the suggested diet only gives her 1,600 calories a day, so that each day she burns up 500 calories from her stored fat. To loose 50,000 calories will take 100 days. There is no instant cure!! The recommended diet will enable a woman to lose just under 1 lb. (0·4 kg.) a week, but she will have to accept that in some weeks she will lose less than in others, because at certain times of the month, usually a week before menstruation, a woman normally retains water. So do not weigh yourself more often than once a week.

OVARIES–REMOVAL

The removal of a woman's ovaries by surgery when she is younger than 45 years is followed by very severe 'menopausal symptoms'. These can be very distressing. In the past, unfortunately, many ovaries were removed unnecessarily by surgeons who had not had a proper training in gynaecology. A gynaecologist who has to operate on a young woman because of pelvic disease will use all his skill to preserve her ovaries. This is possible, even if the ovaries are enlarged by cysts. The cysts can be carefully dissected out of the ovaries, leaving enough ovarian tissue to reconstruct an ovary which functions well. Very occasionally a woman younger than 45 years develops ovarian cancer; in this disease it is essential that both ovaries are removed, but treatment with small tablets of oestrogen hormone, given by mouth, will reduce or eliminate menopausal symptoms.

'PREMENSTRUAL TENSION' AND 'PELVIC CONGESTION'

In the few days before menstruation many women develop 'premenstrual tension'. This is due to water being retained abnormally in the body under the influence of the female sex hormones. The woman may notice that her breasts become tender and swollen; that she gets 'bags' under her eyes; and that her abdomen feels bloated. Some women develop migraine at this time, whilst others become constipated. Even more annoying, a woman may become irritable with her husband and family, occasionally depressed, sometimes sleepy, and prone to headaches. These conditions are fairly common, and if they are severe can be treated by giving tablets which encourage her to get rid of the retained water and consequently to pass more urine, and occasionally by prescribing tranquillizers until menstruation relieves the symptoms.

PELVIC CONGESTION. In 'pelvic congestion' certain symptoms of premenstrual tension persist throughout the menstrual cycle, but are usually more severe in the days before menstruation. The patient complains of feelings of pressure in the pelvis, backache, and vague feelings of being unwell. Often these women have heavier periods. The symptoms are thought to be due to congestion of the pelvic organs with blood, and this in turn is due to emotional stress. Although many women with these symptoms feel that an operation to remove the uterus would help, and many doctors perform a hysterectomy, the results are not good. The best treatment is for the woman to try and resolve her emotional problems, seeking the help of a sympathetic gynaecologist, or a psychiatrist when necessary.

PROLAPSE

If the tissues which support the vagina and uterus are abnormally stretched during childbirth, or if a tear of the perineum is not repaired, the woman may later experience symptoms of prolapse, or what is often called a 'fallen womb'. The prolapse may involve a weakness of the front wall of the vagina–called a *cystocele*; a weakness of the back wall of the vagina, usually associated with damage also to the tissues between the vagina and the rectum–called a *rectocele*; or a weakness of the supports of the womb, which is a *uterine prolapse*.

The weakness of the front vaginal wall–or cystocele–may make a bulge or lump which can be felt just inside the vagina or at its entrance when the patient strains. Unless it is associated with bladder symptoms such as frequency of urination, infection of the urine as shown by laboratory tests, or unless it is very marked, surgery is not required.

The weakness of the back vaginal wall, particularly if there is also an unrepaired tear of the perineum, makes the entrance to the vagina larger, and a lump may be felt there on straining. Once again, unless it causes symptoms, treatment is not really required.

The prolapse of the womb itself only needs treatment if the cervix projects from the vagina, or if the symptoms of 'something falling out' become annoying. The womb normally 'drops' a little down the vagina when the pressure in the abdomen is increased, as in straining to open the bowels, and the cervix may be felt just inside the vaginal entrance. So long as the tissues have good tone and a good blood supply, the minor degree of prolapse does not worry the woman; but after the menopause the blood supply is reduced and the tissues become less flexible, so that the prolapse becomes more obvious and symptoms begin. Prolapse of the womb does not cause backache, despite what is believed.

Once a 'prolapse' causes symptoms, treatment is generally surgical. However today, with better obstetric care, severe prolapse is less common, and the big operations of the past are less often required. Since many patients who have small degrees of prolapse do not need treatment at all, the decision to operate should only be made by an experienced gynaecologist.

'RETROVERSION' OF THE WOMB

Normally the womb lies bent forward at an angle of nearly 90° to that of the vagina, and it is able to rotate about an axis at the level of the cervix (Fig. **19/2**). As the bladder fills, it pushes the uterus up and backwards, and if a woman lies on her back her womb may 'tilt backwards'. In 10 per cent of women the womb is normally tilted backwards. The condition is called 'retroversion', and it can

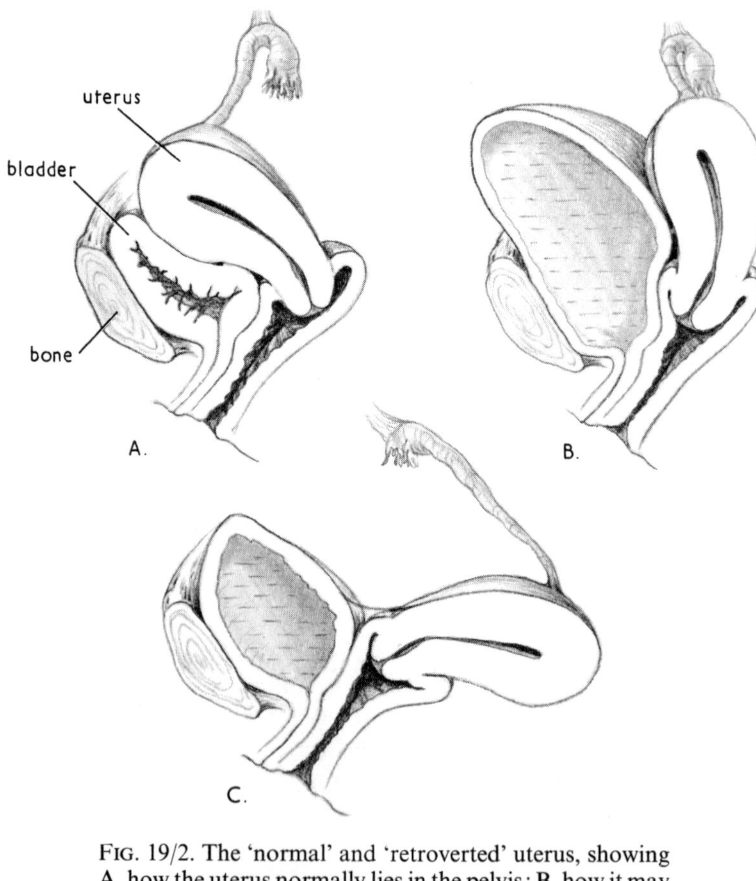

FIG. 19/2. The 'normal' and 'retroverted' uterus, showing A. how the uterus normally lies in the pelvis; B. how it may move when the bladder fills and C. a 'retroverted' uterus

occur from time to time in women whose uterus normally lies bent forwards, or anteverted. In the past an amazing variety of gynaecological disorders have been attributed to retroversion of the uterus; these included backache, sterility, vaginal discharge, pelvic pain, headaches, constipation, diminished sexual desire, frequency of urination and 'wind'! The many operations devised to 'correct' the retroversion made the doctors rich, but did little to cure the patient's symptoms which, although temporarily relieved, returned after a while. Retroversion is often called 'twisting' of the womb by doctors who try to explain the condition to their patients. This is a bad term, for a twisted womb implies a dangerous condition which needs careful surgery for correction, when all that has happened is that the uterus has *tilted* backwards, a quite normal event.

It is now known that unless the womb is *fixed* in the retroverted position by infection or endometriosis, it is of no importance that it is retroverted, as it causes none of the symptoms attributed to it, and there is no need for an operation or the use of supporting 'pessaries' which were once popular.

'TROUBLE WITH THE WATER'

A singularly distressing complaint, which most often occurs after the age of 40, is an 'irritable bladder'. This is not the medical term, and the condition is more properly called 'urgency incontinence', but in fact the patient complains of an 'irritable bladder'. In most cases the woman finds that she gets the urge to empty her bladder at very frequent intervals, and the urge may be stimulated by coughing, jolting in a bus or car, or something of that nature. Once she begins to urinate, she has to go on until her bladder is empty, but because she passes urine so frequently, she only voids a small amount of urine each time. Occasionally an irritable bladder is due to some disorder such as infection, but in most cases it is due to an emotional upset which shows itself in this way. The doctor will have to make tests to decide what is the cause, as only then can he give treatment. This is always medical, and surgery is not needed.

There is another kind of urination trouble which may inconvenience a woman. In this a tiny amount of urine escapes and soils the underclothes whenever the patient strains, coughs or laughs. The woman may be young or old, but has usually given birth to one or more children. The condition is called 'stress incontinence' because the loss of urine occurs after a stress or strain. It can occur whether the bladder is full or apparently empty. The doctor has to differentiate this condition very carefully from urgency incontinence, because the more annoying forms of stress incontinence do require surgical treatment. The lesser forms, when the loss of urine only occurs occasionally, can be treated by the patient doing exercises to strengthen the muscles which support the vagina and the urethra – the short tube connecting the bladder to the outside. The exercises consist of tightening the muscle of the 'tail' without using the abdominal muscles. I describe this as 'trying to make the anus, or back-passage opening, touch the mouth'. A woman can do the exercises in any free moment, and should aim at doing them at least one hundred times a day.

URINARY TRACT INFECTION

The urinary tract starts at the kidney, continues as the tube (the ureter) between the kidney and the bladder, expands as the bladder and then goes on as the tube (the urethra) between the bladder and the outside. Infection of the urinary tract is usually due to the spread of bacteria from the outside up along the urethra to infect the bladder (called 'cystitis'), and then in most cases up the ureter to infect the kidney (called 'pyelonephritis'). Because a woman has a shorter urethra than a man, she is more likely to develop infection of the bladder. Luckily in most cases this is of no importance, as the bladder itself kills the bacteria, so that the urine is sterile, but it appears that about 5 per cent of girls and women harbour active bacteria in their bladders. These bacteria may cause infection at any time, but especially during the first weeks of marriage ('honeymoon cystitis'), and in pregnancy. It is thought that the movement of the penis against the urethra and bladder which occurs in sexual intercourse stimulates the bacteria to grow, and in pregnancy the urine tends to stagnate in the bladder.

The symptoms of urinary tract infection are frequency of urination, and painful urination especially towards the end of voiding. If infection has involved the kidney, backache in the kidney area, fever and chills develop.

If a woman develops these symptoms, she should consult a

doctor so that he may have the urine examined for bacteria, and prescribe treatment. Untreated urinary tract infection can lead to kidney damage.

VAGINAL DISCHARGE

In several investigations it has been found that the most common reason for a woman to see a doctor is that she has a vaginal discharge. Vaginal discharges are of several kinds, some requiring treatment and others being perfectly normal and of no importance. To understand them it must be remembered that the vagina, like the uterus, is part of the genital tract, and that the tissues which make up the tract are very strongly influenced by the female sex hormones, oestrogen and progesterone. Oestrogen stimulates the tissues to mature, and progesterone further develops them. This is most obvious in pregnancy, but changes occur in the lining tissues of the vagina, the cervix, as well as the uterus during each menstrual cycle. The changes caused by oestrogen make the cells lining the cervix secrete a thin, slightly sticky mucus, and this is most marked midway between the periods. The cells which make up the lining of the vagina are arranged rather like bricks making up a wall. The top cells are thin and large. These top cells are constantly shed into the vagina, rather like leaves falling off a tree; in fact, they are said to 'exfoliate'–which means just that. In the vagina they are acted upon by the helpful bacteria which normally live there, to produce a weak acid. This acid–called lactic acid–prevents dangerous bacteria from growing in the vagina. The vaginal cells and the cervical mucus add to the vaginal discharge. As well, some fluid seeps between the cells of the vaginal wall to join the secretions in the vagina. This seepage is increased during sexual excitement, during anxiety, when sexual frustration occurs, or if the woman is ill or emotionally upset.

It can be seen that the quantity of the normal vaginal secretions can vary very considerably and still be quite normal, just as the quantity of secretions in the mouth (the saliva) varies very considerably. The secretions not only keep the vagina moist, which is desirable, but keep it clean. However, from time to time the increased secretions may stain the woman's panties and cause her concern. Usually, if the discharge is not irritating, it is of little importance and treatment is not required. Indeed, in certain conditions, such as when taking a sequential oral contraceptive, an increased vaginal discharge may be expected to occur. However, if the amount of the discharge is annoying, the woman should consult her doctor. He will take a swab sample of the discharge and look at it under the microscope before prescribing treatment. This non-irritant vaginal discharge, which may or may not have 'an odour', is called leukorrhoea–or the 'whites'–but it is bad to give it a name, as it immediately becomes something abnormal in most people's minds, whereas in fact it is quite normal.

Irritating vaginal discharges

If the discharge causes itching and pain in the vagina and around its opening in the vulva, the condition is generally due to some disease and certainly requires investigation. Two main kinds of disorder can cause the trouble. The first, and most common, is when a tiny living organism (called a trichomonad) gets into the vagina. This organism is composed of a single cell, and has a powerful tail (Fig. **19/3**). How it gets into the vagina of about one

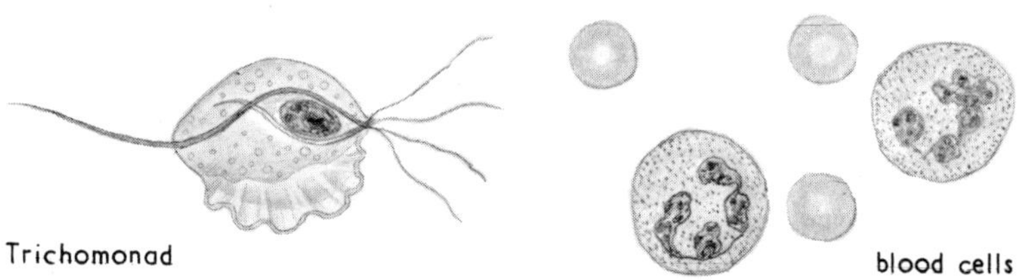

FIG. 19/3. Trichomonads seen under the microscope

woman in every three is unknown, but there is a lot of evidence that it is transmitted during sexual intercourse. In most women it lives quietly in the velvet-like lining of the vagina, and causes no symptoms; in most men it lives quietly in the urinary tract tube within the penis. But in some women, for some unknown reason, it can cause a severe vaginal and vulval itch. The diagnosis is made after the doctor has taken a specimen from the vagina and looked at it under a microscope, when the organism can be seen wriggling about, its tail thrashing. Treatment is easy and effective, and is by giving tablets which can be swallowed. Since the husband often harbours the trichomonads without knowing it, treatment should be given to him as well as to his wife.

The second, less common, cause of an itchy vagina is when a fungus gets into the vagina and grows there. This is more common in pregnancy and if the woman has diabetes, as the fungus – called Candida albicans – prefers a sugary, warm atmosphere in which to grow. But fungal infection can occur in other women. The vaginal discharge can be quite heavy, the itch intolerable, and the woman is in considerable discomfort. The husband may also be infected and have an itchy penis. Once again, the diagnosis is made by examining a specimen of the discharge under a microscope. Treatment is given by inserting special tablets high into the vagina over a three-week period, and by applying an ointment to the skin of the vulva. The husband should also use the ointment on his penis.

Of course, other conditions can cause a vaginal discharge, and will be diagnosed after examination by a doctor. One of the most important is a discharge due to gonorrhoea, and this is considered in the next section. Another is the so-called cervical 'erosion'.

Cervical 'erosion'

As noted previously, the lining of the vagina is built up of layers of cells, rather like a wall is built up of bricks, and the same arrangement of cells covers the cervix where it pokes into the upper part of the vagina. However, a sudden change occurs at the edge of the canal leading through the cervix. The cells which line this are a single layer thick. They are large and very active in secreting mucus. During puberty, and again in a first pregnancy, the exact position of the change from the flat wall-like cells of the vaginal part of the cervix to the tall single mucus-secreting cells of the cervical canal moves, and in many women it moves outwards. This means that the tall cells now appear around the entrance to the canal to look like lips (Fig. **19/4**). The same effect can be obtained if you close your mouth and draw in your lips. Your mouth now appears as a slit ringed by pink skin. If you now pout your lips, your mouth is ringed by red lip mucous membrane.

In the past, the 'pouting' of the cells of the cervical canal was called an 'erosion' or an 'ulcer' because doctors believed it was

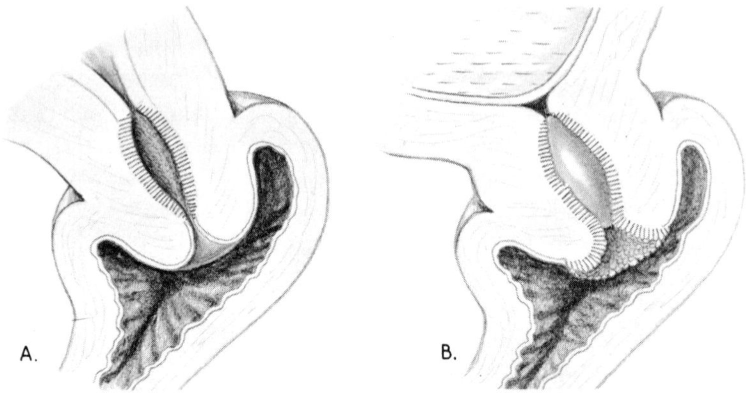

FIG. 19/4. The junction between the lining cells of the cervical canal and those of the cervix move in pregnancy

abnormal. And, of course, it is *not* an ulcer. The treatment of the 'ulcer' was to burn it by applying a cautery stick or by burning it using an electric cautery. It is now known that such treatment is usually unnecessary, and indeed is only needed if at childbirth the mouth of the cervical canal is torn or damaged. However, even in these cases treatment should be withheld for at least six months after childbirth, as the 'pouting' often disappears. Only if it persists beyond this time and leads to a marked vaginal discharge, is cautery needed. The stick cautery is quite useless, and only the electric cautery is of value. The treatment can be given in the doctor's office, but is often best done in hospital under an anaesthetic.

After the cautery of the cervix, the woman will notice that she has a greatly increased quantity of vaginal discharge, often dirty-looking with streaks of blood in the first few days. The discharge is due to the burned area being shed as the cells beneath it make a new lining and push off the old one. The discharge may last for 4 to 6 weeks, but this is normal. At the end of this time, the doctor usually wants to see the patient once again, so that he may inspect the cervix to see how well it has healed.

Vaginal odours

The vagina is self-cleansing, but some women notice that there may be a 'smell'. It is quite normal for the vulva and vagina to have a faint 'odour', just as does the penis, and in general it is quite unnoticeable to other people. However, some women *imagine* that the vaginal odour can be detected by all the passers-by. This is not true, and in fact if a woman bathes each day, the odour will be undetectable. However, the belief of a 'vaginal odour' is encouraged by manufacturers who sell deodorants for 'personal, intimate, feminine freshness', or to give the woman 'day-long protection and a new sense of feminine security'. These sales gimmicks work by making a woman who does not use deodorants feel less feminine and less secure, and appeal to her need for hygiene. In fact, a deodorant works by adding a different smell – usually a perfume – which vanishes in a short time, but inspires the belief that it persists. In general, then, the average girl or woman who bathes each day has no need for vaginal deodorants, but if she wants to spend her money on these unnecessary gimmicks, they are readily (if fairly expensively) available.

Vaginal douching

The use of the vaginal douche for purposes of feminine 'hygiene', to 'remove odour', and immediately after sexual intercourse is a peculiarly American habit, which in recent years has waned in popularity. The idea that the vagina needed washing out was based of false premises, and was connected with the American obsession for personal cleanliness. Whilst it is reasonable and proper to wash the body, including the vulva, daily to remove the accumulated secretions of the sweat glands, the logic of washing out the vagina is less certain. This is because of the vagina's ability to 'cleanse' itself by producing lactic acid. The conclusion must be that there is in general no need for a woman to use vaginal douches, and in fact there is every reason to avoid them.

VENEREAL DISEASES

Venereal diseases are defined as diseases which are transmitted by sexual intercourse. The two traditional venereal diseases have a long history. Gonorrhoea is known to have occurred since ancient times, but syphilis was only introduced in Europe and Asia with the return of Columbus's ships and sailors from the voyage of discovery of America. Except in very rare and special circumstances, the diseases are only spread by sexual intercourse. This means that if a woman develops either syphilis or gonorrhoea, she has caught it from a man who previously caught it from a woman, and so on back in time. Obviously, if promiscuity is reduced, and if men and women fornicate with few partners, or do not have sexual intercourse except with the partner they propose to marry or until after marriage, the spread of the diseases would be limited. Unfortunately, from the viewpoint of control of infection, this ideal situation does not exist, and recently in all countries there has been a rising incidence of the venereal diseases. In part this is due to increasing sexual permissiveness, but in part to the involvement of many thousands of young men in the Vietnam and other wars. When you are young, alone, frustrated and in danger, sexual intercourse is a release, although with a prostitute it is a certain way of catching syphilis or gonorrhoea. The germs which cause the two diseases have become very resistant to treatment, and a partly-treated male can infect several women, who in turn infect other males.

Gonorrhoea is the more frequent disease, and in woman can have disastrous effects if not treated quickly and adequately. The symptoms are usually all too obvious: within five days of being infected during sexual intercourse, the girl complains of a discharge from her urethra, and pain and frequency on passing urine. As well she usually develops a heavy vaginal discharge. At this stage the disease is completely curable, but if it is not treated at once, the bacteria will spread upwards through the cavity of the uterus to infect the oviducts, rendering the girl sterile, and unable to have children. The diagnosis is made by careful examination of specimens of discharge taken from the urethra, from the vagina and from the cervix. Treatment is urgent, and must be followed out completely.

Syphilis is a more serious condition, and is often hard to detect in a woman. Usually within 14 to 28 days, but sometimes as long as 90 days after sexual intercourse with an infected man, a small sore appears on one of the lips of the vulva (the labia). It is relatively painless, but the labium may become swollen and tender. Usually the sore persists for a few weeks, unless treatment is given, and then disappears. Unfortunately in some infected women the sore, or chancre, may not develop on the labium, but upon the cervix where it is undetected, and only when a faint pink, spotty rash appears on the chest, back and arms does the girl seek medical advice. The rash, if due to syphilis, persists for several weeks, so that a rash which appears and fades over a few days is not due to the disease. However, if a girl develops a pink, spotty rash which lasts for more than 10 days, and if she has had sexual intercourse with more than one man, or even with a man she knows well, it would be wise for her to have a blood test done.

Syphilis carries two dangers to woman unless it is treated. The immediate danger is that when she becomes pregnant, her baby is very likely to develop syphilis whilst still in the womb; the long-term danger is that untreated syphilis causes damage to the nervous system and may lead to madness.

Neither of these two disasters need occur if treatment is obtained early. Syphilis is curable, although the treatment required must be followed with great care, and the patient requires to have her blood tested at intervals for several years.

VULVAL ITCHINESS

The skin of the vulval area is particularly sensitive to stimuli, and an itching vulva is a fairly common complaint. If the itch is sufficiently annoying for the woman to seek medical help, she will require proper investigation, as a vulval itch has several causes. Most commonly, it is due to vaginal infection and discharge, or to general diseases such as diabetes or general skin conditions; but in a fairly large number of cases, the itch is an outward sign of an inward frustration, usually of a sexual nature. The itch makes the woman scratch, especially at night; scratching irritates the vulval skin, which causes further itchiness, which causes further scratching, and so on. After careful investigation, the doctor can make a diagnosis and can offer treatment. In this three things need to be known:

firstly, treatment is medical not surgical; secondly, the longer the woman has had the itch before seeking help, the longer it takes to cure; and thirdly, if any cause is found it needs proper treatment, and the patient cannot hope for instant cure. She must be patient and rely upon her doctor.

CHAPTER 20

An ounce of prevention . . .

As most of the diseases which previously killed people in infancy, childhood and adolescence have come under control, the cancers which afflict older people have come under increasing investigation and study. Calculations have been made which show that a woman has a 5 per cent chance of developing cancer of the breast; a 2·7 per cent chance of developing a cancer of the gut; a 2·3 per cent chance of developing cancer of the cervix of the womb; and a 2·0 per cent chance of developing a cancer of the body of the womb. This means that of every 100 females born, 5 will develop cancer of the breast, and 4 will develop cancer of the womb at some time before death. Apart from cancer of the gut, cancer of the genital organs (in which I include the breast) are the most common cancers found in women.

The only sure way to control cancer and to prevent it from killing its host, is to detect it before it has grown very far. Women are luckier than men in this respect, for the breasts and the womb are relatively easily accessible for examination, provided the patient attends for regular periodic check-ups.

The American Cancer Association, in an admirable series of booklets, emphasizes the importance of early detection of cancer, and advises women to consult their doctor immediately if any of the following symptoms or signs appear:

1. Any sore that does not heal quickly, especially about the mouth.
2. Any unusual bleeding or discharge from any natural body opening.
3. Any painless lump, especially in the breasts, lips, tongue or soft tissues.
4. Any persistent indigestion or unexplained weight loss.
5. Any persistent hoarseness or cough or difficulty in swallowing.
6. Any unexplained change in normal bowel habits.

This advice is sensible and timely, and if women followed it, would lead to a reduction in the deaths which occur from cancer. The three signs which may indicate a cancer of the breast or genital tract are: (1) any painless lump in the breast, (2) any unusual bleeding or discharge from the vagina, and (3) a sore or ulcer on the vulva which does not heal quickly. Only by early detection and proper treatment can the fatal outcome of cancer be prevented. An ounce of prevention is far more valuable than a pound of attempted cure!

CANCER OF THE BREAST

The earliest sign of cancer of the breast is a small, rounded painless lump. Not every lump found in the breast is due to cancer, but every lump is suspect. For this reason, regular self-examination of the breasts is recommended as described in Chapter 18. This self-examination should be supplemented by regular visits to the doctor each year, so that he may also palpate the woman's breasts. At present investigations are being undertaken to see if more sophisticated methods using instruments will detect possible breast cancer earlier. X-ray examination of the breasts (called mammography) has proved only partially helpful, but a method using heat-rays may be better. Time alone will tell, and in the meantime every woman should routinely perform self-examination of the breasts, at monthly intervals preferably after her menstrual period in the reproductive years of life, but equally at monthly intervals after the menopause.

CANCER OF THE CERVIX OF THE WOMB

It is unfortunate that by the time cancer of the cervix is visible to the naked eye, it is so far advanced that no matter what treatment is given, one woman in every two will be dead within five years. But if it is detected before it is visible, the disease is 100 per cent curable.

The method used for detection is to take a sample of the cells which cover the cervix. This sample is then fixed in alcohol, and sent to a special cytological laboratory where it is stained with Papanicolaou's stain and examined for 'abnormal cells'. The specimen is called a 'Pap-smear', because Dr. Papanicolaou, who worked in New York, first pointed out that early cancer cells of the cervix were less sticky than normal cells, and were shed (or exfoliated) more readily into the vagina. To take the specimen the doctor inserts a small instrument, called a speculum, into the vagina and looks at the cervix. He then takes a 'scraping' from the cervix using a wooden spatula, similar to that used for depressing the tongue when he wants to look down the throat. He also takes a sample from the upper vagina, and from the canal of the cervix. The whole procedure is quite painless, and the doctor takes the opportunity to do a pelvic examination at the same time to be sure that there is nothing wrong with the uterus or the ovaries.

The pelvic examination and 'Pap-smear' should be made twice in the year after the first attendance, and then every one to three years until the woman is 65. The first test is often made when a girl becomes pregnant for the first time, and should certainly be made on every woman who has had sexual intercourse once she reaches the age of 25.

There is evidence that cancer of the cervix is related in some way to sexual intercourse, as the disease is very rare in nuns, and is found most frequently amongst women who have had sexual intercourse in their teens, often with several partners, and have had their first baby before the age of 20. However, by no means every woman with cancer of the cervix has this history. Unfortunately, too, the disease appears to occur more frequently amongst women of the lower socio-economic groups, or more exactly amongst poorer, less educated women. These women are the very ones who do not seek medical care and are reluctant to have routine 'Pap-smears' performed.

Any campaign to eliminate cancer of the cervix must include an attempt to get every woman in the area – especially the poor – to have pelvic examinations and 'Pap-smears' performed at regular intervals.

The smear is looked at down a microscope by a trained technician and 'abnormal' smears are checked by a qualified doctor. Of every 1,000 smears examined, about 20 will show 'abnormal' cells, and 3 of these will be really worrying. If 'abnormal' cells are found, a further smear is done, and a specimen is taken from the cervix. This specimen may be taken with a tiny punch, after looking at the cervix with a special magnifying instrument called a colposcope. If this instrument is used, the patient does not need an anaesthetic, and the whole procedure can be done without admitting her to hospital. In other cases, the patient does require admission, and a larger piece of the cervix is cut out. This is like coring out an apple, and is called 'conization'. The cervix is stitched and heals easily.

If the pieces of tissue or the 'cone' show very early cancer, treatment is given. Usually if the patient wants to have more children, the cone is sufficient treatment, but if she has completed her family, a hysterectomy is performed. In either case, she will have to continue to attend her doctor after the operation at regular intervals, for further 'Pap-smears'. If the tissues show more advanced cancer – and only a very few do – the woman will have to have a much more extensive regimen of radiation therapy or surgery.

Only by regular pelvic examinations and 'Pap-smears' will cancer of the cervix be eliminated. Every woman should therefore make sure that she has this simple, painless test done at regular intervals from the time of her first pregnancy or the age of 25, whichever is the earlier, to the age of 65 or later.

CANCER OF THE BODY OF THE WOMB

This is a little less common than cancer of the cervix, and usually occurs when the woman is older. In fact, it is most often found in women aged 50 to 60. Unfortunately 'smear' tests do not readily detect cancer of the body of the womb, and consequently the doctor has to rely on symptoms. Any woman who develops irregular bleeding after the age of 35 should see her doctor. The bleeding is most likely to be due to hormonal changes, but it may be the first sign of cancer of the womb. An even more sinister sign is bleeding which occurs *after* the menopause. However scanty the bleeding is, the woman must see her doctor at once so that he can arrange for a diagnostic curettage if he thinks this is necessary. Luckily cancer of the body of the womb grows very slowly, so that if the woman follows this advice, it is generally curable.

CANCER OF THE VULVA

This is a relatively rare form of cancer found principally in old women and preceded by a vulval itch, usually of long duration. Any elderly woman who has an itchy vulva which persists should seek medical attention. In order to exclude early cancer of the vulval skin, the doctor may need to take tiny pieces of skin. The procedure is done under a local anaesthetic and does not disturb the patient.

CANCER OF THE OVARIES

About 5 per cent of all cancers which develop in women are cancers of the ovaries, and these account for 10 per cent of cancers of the genital tract. In all cases the first sign is enlargement of the ovary, which can be detected on pelvic examination; but 95 per cent of ovarian enlargement is non-cancerous, and only 5 per cent of the enlargements are due to cancer. Cancer is more likely to occur after the age of 40, and particularly likely after the menopause.

Since the growth is silent and slow, the disease is difficult to detect, and the only way is for women aged 40 and over to have periodic pelvic examinations to detect ovarian enlargement. The finding of an enlarged ovary at this age is an indication for surgery, so that the tumour may be removed and examined under the microscope.

CHAPTER 21

Not the end of life

At a time which is quite variable and individual for a woman, the remaining egg follicles in the ovary (numbering about 8,000) begin to disappear. This strange and unexplained event occurs some time between the 45th and 55th year of life. The changes are not abrupt, and there is a gradual transition from the normal ovarian activity of the reproductive years, to the relatively inactive ovary of the menopausal years.

The first change in the sequence of events which culminates in the cessation of menstruation, or the menopause, is that the egg follicles in the ovary become increasingly less sensitive to stimulation by the hormones of the pituitary. In addition, there is a change in the quantity of the two pituitary hormones–FSH and LH–which have stimulated the growth of some follicles each month since adolescence. These two changes mean that fewer egg follicles are stimulated, and consequently reduced, but variable, amounts of oestrogen are released during each menstrual cycle. For this reason the lining of the uterus is less satisfactorily stimulated, and the menstrual flow becomes less regular and predictable. The quantity of the blood lost gets less, and the interval between the menstrual periods is usually increased. The co-ordinated control of menstruation which has been so effective since adolescence is getting out of gear, as the controlling glands 'unwind' into a quieter phase of life.

As the months pass fewer egg follicles are stimulated and the amount of oestrogen secreted by them diminishes still further, until eventually the menstrual periods cease altogether. The menopause has arrived.

Of course, the sequence may not be so smooth. Some women develop heavy bleeding episodes, as sudden surges of oestrogen occur, followed by long intervals when the menstrual periods are absent. For this is a time of hormonal turbulence, only slightly less than that which occurred at puberty. The whole period of change is more properly called the climacteric, or 'change of life', whilst the ceasing of menstrual periods is called the menopause; but the term menopause is commonly used for both events.

THE CHANGES IN THE BODY

All the changes which occur are due to altered hormone secretion, and result from a fall in oestrogen, an absence of progesterone, and a rise in pituitary hormones. It used to be thought that oestrogen ceased to be produced after the menopause, but now it is known that some continues to be secreted well into old age, but of course the quantity is small.

The main changes which occur in the body of the menopausal woman are due to the diminished secretion of oestrogen. Because oestrogen is most active on the tissues which make up the female genital tract and on the breasts, these are most affected. But because of the continuing but variable amounts of oestrogen secreted, the degree to which they are affected is quite variable.

In the few years before the menopause, the breasts often increase in size as extra fat is deposited; but after the climacteric, this fat is reabsorbed, the gland tissue decreases and the nipples get smaller. These changes take place slowly, but by the age of 65 the breasts are usually flattened and tend to droop. In the same slow manner the uterus, the oviducts and the ovaries become smaller and inactive. The lining wall of the vagina becomes thinner and more easily irritated as the years pass, but this is less likely to occur if sexual intercourse continues to take place. The tissues which surround and support the vagina and the muscles of the floor of the pelvis tend to become flabby, and to lose their elasticity, so that some degree of prolapse may occur. This may be of the front or back wall of the vagina, so that a bulge or lump appears at the vulva when the woman strains; or it may be of the uterus itself, the cervix projecting through the vaginal entrance. The prolapse may look more serious than it really is, because the main lips of the vulva – the labia majora – decrease in size at this time of life. Only a few cases of prolapse give discomfort and need surgery. Most can be left alone. Once again, these changes take place slowly over the years.

MENOPAUSAL SYMPTOMS

More annoying, because they occur earlier and with greater impact, are the 'menopausal symptoms'. Some of these are due to lack of oestrogen, others have not yet been understood completely. In many women the symptoms are minor, and probably no more than one woman in four needs to consult a doctor because of them. Hot flashes, or flushes, may occur, in which a sudden feeling of intense heat sweeps over the body, and a blush spreads over the face and neck. Hot flushes only last a few moments and then go. They tend to recur many times during the day, and are sometimes accompanied by tingling sensations sweeping the body. The hot flushes may be triggered by excitement or emotions, and are the most common menopausal symptoms. They vary in intensity and frequency, but tend to last for months or years, becoming less frequent as time goes by. Almost as common are episodes of sweating, and the onset of irregularities of menstruation. These three symptoms are due to the reduced secretion of oestrogen. Other symptoms which are distressing are depression, insomnia, fatigue, headache and skin changes, but the cause of these is not understood.

PSYCHOLOGICAL CHANGES

Just as the waxing turbulent tides of hormones and the need to adapt to new ways made puberty and adolescence a difficult time, some women find that the waning tides of hormones and the need to adapt to them makes the menopause a difficult time. It is very difficult for doctors to decide if the symptoms of depression, fatigue and insomnia are due to hormonal changes, or to a deep emotional disturbance as the woman looks around and does not like what she sees. Her children are growing up, or have already left the family home; her youthful hopes and desires have dissipated into a routine 'suburban' life; her husband appears to have found other interests, leaving her increasingly alone; her friends have similar problems, and constantly complain about them. She sees these changes, she feels that she has missed something, often a great deal, of what she had imagined life had to offer, and she has to adjust to the strange symptoms of the menopause–or strange to her at any rate. The peculiar irregularity of her periods may subconsciously increase the anxiety that her physical and sexual attractions are waning. She is becoming old, and thinks she is rejected; she has reached the 'end of life'. These vividly felt emotions are, of course, only temporary. Psychiatrists have discovered that many women at the menopause pass through three phases before becoming adjusted to their new life. The first is one in which feelings of anxiety and turmoil are most evident. Usually this period is fairly short and merges into a period which may last months, when irritability, depression and other mood changes are common, and the woman feels rejected by everyone. Nothing is right. In time this phase merges into a phase of readjustment, when all the misery of the previous months seems like a bad dream.

WHAT TO DO AT THE CLIMACTERIC

The first thing for a woman to remember is that the strange feelings which she has are temporary, and that adjustment will come in due course. Women who have interests outside the home find it easier to adjust; but women whose outlook is confined to the house, the backyard, the immediate neighbours and the television set often have problems.

Careful investigations in the U.S.A. and in Britain have shown that about two-thirds of women pass through the 'change of life' without any trouble, or with only a little upset. The remaining one-third need help. Help is available from the family doctor, who knows about the woman and her background. He is particularly well suited to offer sympathetic understanding and the reassurance which is so often needed. He is also able to offer mild sedatives if insomnia is the problem; tranquillizers, if mood changes, irritability and depression are present; or hormones if the hot flushes and sweats are causing the woman concern.

Despite what has been written in many women's magazines, not every woman who seeks medical help at this time needs hormone treatment. If menstruation is still regular and normal in amount, hormones are of no help. Only if the flushes are of such severity or frequency as to cause annoyance are hormones helpful. Oestrogen – which is the hormone usually prescribed – in small doses will control flushings, but it will not rejuvenate the skin, make the hair glisten, put a blush on the cheeks or a sparkle in the eye of the menopausal woman. She can do all these things by her attitude to the 'change of life', and by realizing that it is a *change* and not the end of life.

The dose of oestrogen required to control the number of hot flushes differs, and most doctors try to use the smallest dose needed to regulate them in that particular woman. To help the doctor, the patient is asked to make a 'hot flush count'. She counts the number of hot flushes she gets each day, and the doctor increases or decreases the dose of oestrogen so that she gets no more than five hot flushes a day. This is 'tailoring' the drug to the patient, and is the best way of controlling the symptoms; but sometimes because the patient is impatient or unable to co-operate, the doctor may prescribe 'the Pill' to control hot flushes. This treatment is effective but more expensive, and the woman, of course, will get a return of her periods.

SEXUAL INTERCOURSE AFTER THE MENOPAUSE

Sexual responsiveness is unaltered by the 'change of life' in 60 per cent of women, 20 per cent have increased sexual urges, and in 20 per cent sexual needs are diminished. Since after the menopause there is no fear of pregnancy, a woman's sexual urge may be increased, and this may improve the relationship between herself and her husband. The fact is that the sexual urge is not related to sex hormone production at or after the menopause. Some women remain desirous of, and anxious for, sexual intercourse well into old age, whilst others are not concerned if sexual intercourse is avoided for many months. Studies in America have shown that women retain their sex potential longer than men, and that 7 out of every 10 couples are sexually active after the age of 60, some continuing into their eighties. The main reason for stopping sexual intercourse is ill health, usually of the husband.

POSTMENOPAUSAL BLEEDING

In the years after the menopause, a few women notice that they have a scanty, or more profuse, bloody discharge coming from the vagina. This is an urgent reason for going to consult their doctor. The bleeding may be unimportant, due to the use of oestrogens (which can cause bleeding), or to a vaginal irritation, but in some cases it is caused by cancer of the womb. It is essential to see the doctor as soon as possible after bleeding is discovered. He will examine the woman and almost certainly do a diagnostic curettage and take a 'Pap-smear', so that he may be quite certain that cancer is not present.

GETTING FAT

A woman's weight depends on three things: the disposition to fatness she has inherited from her parents; the amount of food and drink she consumes; and the amount of energy she uses for her activities. She can not alter her disposition to fatness (and everybody tends to put on a little weight as the years go by), but she can control the other two factors. If she obtains more energy from food and drink than she uses in her daily tasks, the excess will be converted into fat and stored. At the time of the 'change of life' women tend to eat more and to do less, so that their weight increases. Women can avoid excessive weight gain during and after the menopause if they are careful about what they eat, and remember to keep on exercising themselves. This does not mean that the woman needs to do special exercises, although these often help, but that she gardens, goes for walks, plays golf or swims, depending on her inclinations. There is a tendency for women at this time of life to do less housework than formerly, as there is less to do now the family is grown up and helps; to go to more morning tea or coffee parties; to eat cakes more often; and in general to sit around, sometimes thinking, sometimes just sitting. This inertness is a great contributor to the weight gain which occurs at the 'change of life'. It can be avoided if a woman puts her mind to it. Obesity is discussed further in Chapter 19.

'A PILL A DAY KEEPS ILLNESS AT BAY'

Recently, particularly in the U.S.A., there has been considerable discussion about the value of continuing oestrogen tablets long after the need for them for contraception, or to cope with the hot flushes of the climacteric, has passed. Those doctors who believe in oestrogens claim that a daily oestrogen tablet keeps the woman younger and more feminine, prevents the development of heart disease and 'thinning' of the bones, and retards the changes which occur in the tissues of the genital tract. With this belief, they prescribe a daily oestrogen pill until old age. Apart from the expense of such medicines, there is a considerable opinion that they are not necessary. Firstly oestrogens continue to be secreted by certain glands in the body after the menopause, and at least one woman in every two is producing sufficient to keep her genital tract tissues supple and well-developed. Secondly, there is no evidence that oestrogen keeps a woman younger or more feminine, that it prevents heart disease, or that it hinders the 'thinning' of the structure of the bones. But because so much has been written in women's magazines, this matter needs to be discussed further.

Youth and oestrogen

Women (and men!) have for centuries sought the elixir of youth – a drug which would keep them young for longer. Sensational claims have been made from time to time, that this or that drug delayed the onset of ageing, and more particularly rejuvenated sexual vigour. All of them are fraudulent. In the 1920s it was claimed that 'monkey glands' helped. More recently a secret formula made in Rumania, and known to contain a local anaesthetic, procaine, amongst other ingredients, and an extract of the queen bee, has been claimed to be a potent rejuvenator. None of them have fulfilled their claims, nor can the more sophisticated method of injections of fetal cells developed in Switzerland be said to be effective, at least not when looked at scientifically. The suggestion that oestrogen tablets taken daily will enable a woman to retain her youth is equally fallacious. There is no 'Venus Pill' which will keep a woman eternally youthful. Oestrogen will improve the character of the lining tissues of the uterus and vagina if they are defective, but it will do no more. It will not get rid of wrinkles, eliminate a double chin, a sagging breast or an obese abdomen. It will not restore youth. The real hope for women who are growing old is to adjust to the menopausal years, to keep good physical and mental health, to avoid over-eating and under-exercising, and to cultivate new and challenging interests.

Heart disease and oestrogens

For a while it was thought that oestrogen tablets would delay or reduce heart disease, as it had been found that women under the age of 40, who presumably secreted a good amount of oestrogen, had 20 times less risk of developing heart disease compared with men of the same age. Between the ages of 50 and 60, the difference became far less, and the incidence of heart disease in women was only half that of men. This suggested that oestrogens protected the younger woman, and if oestrogen were given in tablet form after the menopause, the protection would continue. However, most of the evidence from carefully conducted research shows that this is not so, and the most effective way to prevent heart attacks is not for post-menopausal women to take oestrogen tablets, but to avoid overeating and to keep exercising. A daily swim, or a walk, is a far better preventive of heart disease than an oestrogen pill.

Osteoporosis and oestrogens

Thinning of the bone structure, or osteoporosis, is a strange condition which disables about one woman in every five who is aged more than 65. It occasionally occurs in younger women who have had their ovaries surgically removed before the age of 40. The bones of the back (the vertebrae) are first affected and collapse, so that severe backache and later a decrease in height occur. Because of these findings, it was suggested that the condition was due to a lack of oestrogen, but this failed to explain why men, who have very little oestrogen, did not develop the disease more often. It is unlikely that a lack of oestrogen is the cause, so that a daily oestrogen pill will not prevent the disease, although *large* doses of oestrogen together with calcium improves the lot of the woman who develops osteoporosis. A far better preventive measure is to make sure that the diet contains sufficient calcium, and that the woman takes sufficient exercise.

Oestrogens and statistics

The further myth about oestrogens and ageing is based on false statistics. It is known that 75 years ago the life expectancy of women was only 50 years. This meant that at birth the average woman might expect to live 50 years. Today the life expectancy is 74. This observation suggested that 75 years ago women were born, grew up, had children, reached the menopause and died–'exploding like sky-rockets without trace' as one writer has said. Today, however, women live longer, and have twenty or more years of life after the menopause without the oestrogen 'support' which had existed earlier. Therefore, it was said oestrogen tablets were needed to help women 'resist the ageing process' and 'to make the postmenopausal woman's world a better place'–as the pharmaceutical companies who sell oestrogens claim in their advertisements.

Alas, the statistics quoted so often are false. The increase in life expectancy has occurred because the deaths in infancy, childhood and adolescence from infectious diseases have been greatly reduced. In 1900 a woman who reached the age of 25 could expect to live until she was 68. Today she may expect to live until she is 74, so that the difference is not all that great. There are, of course, more older women alive today because there are more people in the world, and because fewer children and girls die before they reach adult life. Today about 10 per cent of women are aged 65 or over, and in the year 2,000, the same proportion is expected. This is indeed a considerable proportion of the population. Their needs for recreation, for exercise, for social intercourse, for a place in society and in the family will require careful consideration, but to say that in the past women did not live after the menopause is nonsense. Many did, and managed very well without a daily oestrogen tablet!

Oestrogens and the ageing vagina

It is true that if a woman develops a vaginal irritation or finds sexual intercourse painful, the cause may be thinning of the vaginal lining because of deficient oestrogen. This only affects a few postmenopausal women, and is easily corrected by the application into the vagina of a cream containing oestrogen. The use of oestrogen in this way is very sensible and medically correct, whilst its routine use for all women is expensive and ridiculous. It may also be potentially dangerous. There is now some evidence that oestrogens given by mouth or by injection may increase the chance of a woman developing clots in her blood vessels, and as such mishaps are much more common in older women, it is an additional reason for avoiding the routine use of oestrogen tablets.

To be more scientific, some doctors only prescribe oestrogen tablets if a smear taken from the wall of the vagina and examined under a microscope shows a pattern of cells suggesting an oestrogen lack. The approach is more rational, but is still inexact, and it would be better to avoid oestrogens in the postmenopausal years unless there are symptoms which are due to oestrogen deficiency.

GROWING OLD GRACEFULLY

The menopause is only a milestone on a woman's path through life. If she is well adjusted, or becomes well adjusted after receiving medical help, she will pass through the turbulent years, her character unimpaired. She will be ready to meet the excitement and the challenges of the postmenopausal years. Years which can be as full of interest as any other period of life, provided she herself makes sure that they are. She is growing old gracefully. Not ageing, but growing old, for ageing suggests something sinister, the result of unwise or improvident living, and the abuse of the human machine. Growing old begins at the moment of birth, and continues until death. The menopause is but a milestone along the road, and the 'change of life' is not the end of life.

There can be no more appropriate note on which to end a book about 'Everywoman'.

GLOSSARY

Alveoli (pron. al-*vee*-o-li)
The plural of alveolus, which means a small cavity. The outermost parts of the duct system of the breast, where milk is secreted, are called alveoli.

Amenorrhoea (pron. a-men-or-*e*-a)
The absence of menstruation for an interval twice that (or more) of the patient's usual menstrual cycle.

Analgesic
A pain-relieving drug.

Antenatal period
The period between conception and childbirth. Also called the prenatal period.

Aphrodisiac
A drug or substance which increases sexual desire.

Areola (pron. aree-*o*-la)
The brownish-coloured pigmented area which surrounds the nipple.

Bacillus
A small form of life, made up of a single cell shaped like a tiny rod, often called a germ. Germs may be harmful to man, for example the pneumococcus which causes pneumonia, and the streptococcus which causes sore throats; or they may be helpful, as the lacto-bacillus which lives in the vagina.

Coitus (pron. *ko*-it-us)
The act of sexual intercourse, or copulation. The verb is 'to copulate'.

Coitus interruptus
Coitus in which the penis is withdrawn from the vagina before male orgasm, and the semen is ejaculated externally to the vagina.

Conception sac
The embryo (or fetus) contained in the fluid-filled amniotic membranes is called the conception sac.

Copulate
To practise sexual intercourse.

Eclampsia
The occurrence of convulsions or fits in a pregnant woman who has other signs of 'toxaemia of pregnancy'.

Ejaculate
To spurt out. Applied in this context to the spurting out of semen at the time of orgasm.

Embryo (pron. *em*-bry-o)
The product of conception (or conceptus) from the day of fertilization of the egg cell (ovum) by the spermatozoon until the beginning of the 7th week. During this short period almost all of the major structures have formed.

'Eye' of the penis
The part of the end of the penis through which the urinary tube passes to reach the outside.

Fetus (pron. *fee*-tus)
The product of conception from the end of the 7th week until birth, at whatever period of the pregnancy this may be, is called a fetus.

FSH
Follicle-stimulating hormone. The substance secreted by the pituitary gland which lies beneath the brain. This hormone stimulates some of the egg follicles of the ovary to manufacture oestrogen.

Gestagen
A synthetic–man-made–substance which acts in the body in a way similar to the natural hormone, progesterone.

Heterosexual
A person whose sexual affections are directed to a person of the other sex.

Homosexual
A noun (i.e. a person is called a homosexual) or an adjective (i.e. a homosexual act) implying that the object of a person's sexual desire is of the same sex. In slang, the male homosexual is called a fairy, a pansy, a queen or a queer, while a female homosexual is referred to as a dike or a butch. Butch is also used as an adjective to describe a female homosexual who displays outward manifestations of masculinity in behaviour or in dress.

Hormone
A substance which is released from special glands into the blood stream and stimulates other glands or tissues into activity.

Lactation
Suckling. The period when the child is nourished from the breast. It also means the secretion or formation of milk.

Lesbian
A female homosexual.

LH
Luteinising hormone. The second of the pituitary gonadotrophic, or ovary-stimulating, hormones. It converts the cells of the stimulated egg follicle, from which the egg has been expelled by ovulation, to produce the female sex hormone, progesterone. The cells which produce progesterone become bright yellow (for which the Latin word is '*luteus*'), hence luteinising hormone.

Lochia
The discharge from the uterus which lasts for about 4 weeks after childbirth. For the first few days it is profuse and red, later becoming pale and scanty.

Masturbation
The mechanical stimulation, usually with the hands or fingers, of the penis, the clitoris or other erogenous zones of the body leading to orgasm.

Menarche (pron. men-*ar*-kee)
The time of onset of the first menstrual period.

Menstrual cycle
The interval of time from the start of one menstruation (the 'period') to the next. It includes the time during which bleeding occurs and the interval between bleeding episodes.

Oedema (pron. e-*de*ma)
Swelling of the tissues under the skin due to retention of water in these tissues.

Oestrogen (pron. *ee*-strogen)
The female sex hormone manufactured in the ovary, and in pregnancy in the placenta. The word derives from *oestrous*, or heat-making, because the hormone was found to be necessary to bring animals 'on heat'.

Orgasm
Intense excitement occurring at the climax of sexual intercourse culminating in involuntary jerking movement of the pelvis, a feeling of warmth, well-being and release, and followed by a feeling of relaxation. In the male it is accompanied by the ejaculation, or spurting out, of semen from the penis.

Ovum
The egg cell, which has matured and is ready to be expelled from the ovary, is called the ovum.

Penis (pron. *pee*-nis)
The male sexual organ. Normally it lies soft and limp, but during sexual stimulation it becomes erect. Erections may occur spontaneously at night during sleep, after visual stimuli from magazines, from the sight of sexually-desirable girls, or during the preliminaries of love-making. Erection is not under the control of the mind.

Perineum
The area between the thighs which contains the entrance to the vagina and the other female external genitals, which comprise the vulva.

Progesterone (pron. pro-*gest*-erone)
The second main sex hormone produced by the ovaries. The hormone

prepares the body, especially the uterus, for pregnancy. Progesterone is also manufactured by the placenta from its earliest days.

Promiscuity
A girl may be considered promiscuous if she has sexual intercourse with several casual acquaintances over a short period of time. Premarital coitus with a single partner is not promiscuity.

Prophylactic treatment
Treatment, usually with drugs, given to prevent the onset or spread of disease.

Psychosomatic disorder
A condition in which a disturbed emotion manifests itself as a disorder of one part of the body or another, and mimics disease of that part.

Puerperium
The period between childbirth and the time when the uterus has returned to its normal size, which is about 6 to 8 weeks.

Regimen
A specific course or plan of diet or drugs to maintain or improve health, or regulate the way of life.

Renal tract
See Urinary tract.

Reproductive years, or era
The years during which a woman is ovulating, or able to ovulate, and so is able to have a baby. It is the time when the female sex hormones are regularly and rhythmically produced by the ovaries.

Semen
The fluid ejaculated by the male at orgasm. It consists of spermatozoa, mixed with secretions from the ducts and collecting areas which link the testicles (where the spermatozoa are manufactured) and the penis (from which the semen is ejaculated).

'Toxaemia of pregnancy'
A rise of blood pressure occurring in pregnancy, usually associated with the appearance of protein in the urine, is called 'toxaemia of pregnancy'. The term, although convenient, is inexact because no toxin has been found.

Urinary tract

The kidneys, the tubes which connect the kidneys to the bladder (called the ureters), the urinary bladder, and the tube between the bladder and the vulva (called the urethra) form the renal tract. It is also called the urinary tract.

Zona pellucida

The strong translucent outer membrane which surrounds the human egg, rather as the shell surrounds a hen's egg. The zona pellucida only disappears when the fertilized egg reaches the uterine cavity after spending three days in the oviduct.

INDEX

Index